Illustrated Manual of
Fluid and
Electrolyte Disorders

Illustrated Manual of Fluid and Electrolyte Disorders

R. Douglas Collins, M.D., F.A.C.P.

Director, Internal Medicine Residency Program
Pensacola Foundation for Education and Research, Inc. (P.E.P.)
Baptist, Sacred Heart and University Hospitals
Pensacola, Florida

64 Color Illustrations

J. B. Lippincott Company
Philadelphia • *Toronto*

ISBN 0-397-50361 X

Library of Congress Catalog Card Number: 76-6131

Printed in the United States of America

3   5   4   2

Library of Congress Cataloging in Publication Data

Collins, R. Douglas.
    Illustrated manual of fluid and electrolyte disorders.

    Bibliography: p.
    Includes index.
    1. Body fluid disorders.   2. Water-electrolyte balance (Physiology).   I. Title. [DNLM:
1. Water-electrolyte imbalance. WD220 C712i]
RC630.C64   616'.047   76-6131
ISBN 0-397-50361-X

To Fred Zeller

*for the tremendous part he had in
initiating my career as a medical writer*

Preface

Years ago, like most medical students, I became intrigued with the study of fluid and electrolyte disorders. I found many books that adequately described the various alterations in each disorder, but none was accompanied by pictures which allowed a vivid recollection of these alterations and what caused them. The "Gamblegrams"[1] came the closest of any diagrams to being a substantial aid in this task, but they weren't quite what I was looking for. Consequently I began making drawings of my own. Finally I came up with a drawing (Fig. 1) that could be used to explain and recall the alterations in virtually all electrolyte disorders. The reader will note that the intracellular electrolytes are depicted much as they are in the Gamblegram. However, H^+ ion has been added both intracellularly and extracellularly, even though its actual concentration is small (40 ng./L.). In this way a better understanding of pH changes (also shown in the drawing) can be accomplished. In addition plasma protein is added not only because of its buffering effect, but because it is essential in maintaining the proper ratio of plasma volume to the rest of the extracellular fluid. Because changes in blood oxygen content are frequently associated with electrolyte disorders this also has been included. Finally all those organs associated with the homeostasis of the body fluids are included in the drawing (lungs, kidney, sweat glands, etc.). The drawing is a unique feature of this book and one of the principal reasons for its publication!

Of no less importance are the tables in the book. Table 1 presents the symptoms and signs of each electrolyte alteration. The clinician is frequently confronted with electrolyte results, that fail to fit the clinical picture. Table 2 shows the typical electrolyte changes in common clinical disorders. Table 3 presents the differential diagnosis of single electrolyte alterations. However, since most electrolyte changes are multiple Table 4 offers all the possible combinations of electrolyte results that may present together with a differential diagnosis of each set. Table 5 presents typical results obtained from blood gas analysis together with their differential diagnosis to help support or exclude a diagnosis suggested by the other four tables.

Using the basic illustration in Figure 1, three important sections on electrolyte and fluid balance are developed. First the normal metabolism of each element or compound is described. Then the alterations which may occur in various theoretical conditions are described and illustrated. Finally actual clinical entities are described in terms of their pathophysiology, clinical picture, diagnosis and treatment.

A final chapter deals with the basic tools for treatment including formulas to calculate deficits and the various electrolyte solutions that are available.

Of those people who helped make this book possible I particularly want to thank Doctor William McA. Davis for critically reviewing the manuscript and Faye Wilson for her expert typing.

Gail Grist and Sa Smith are responsible for turning my rough sketches into the beautiful illustrations that are such an important part of this book; Gail Grist did the basic color illustration and Sa Smith did the overlays.

R. Douglas Collins, M.D.

Contents

Introduction

This book is geared to one purpose: the diagnosis and treatment of electrolyte disorders encountered in clinical practice. The laboratory returns to the clinician a set of plasma electrolyte values which he must interpret in the light of the clinical picture. These are expressed as an increased, normal or decreased value for each substance. In order to understand these the clinician must first of all understand the normal metabolism (intake, transport, storage, production, excretion, etc.) of each electrolyte. This is discussed and illustrated in Section One. Then he can picture what malfunction in the system caused the excess or deficit. For example if the potassium is elevated is it due to an increased intake or decreased excretion or disturbed regulation?

Section Two presents a discussion of what an excess or deficit of water, H^+ ions and each electrolyte individually does to the rest of the system. This gives the clinician an understanding of the clinical and laboratory features of individual alterations in electrolytes. Diseases usually result in combinations of electrolyte alterations. However, the combinations will be better understood if what happens during the individual alterations is examined first.

Section Three shows how to apply the material learned in Section One and Two to formulating the diagnosis. In Table 1 important clinical data (skin turgor, urine outputs, etc.) are described. Table 2 shows the combination of electrolyte abnormalities in the most common clinical disorders. Frequently the clinician can get an immediate diagnosis of his problem by looking at this table. Table 3 gives the differential diagnosis of individual electrolyte alterations. This table should be consulted when only one electrolyte in the report is abnormal.

Table 4 gives the differential diagnosis of all the possible abnormal combinations that a clinician may encounter. When a laboratory error is the only logical explanation, this is noted. If Table 2 does not give a combination consistent with the laboratory report Table 4 must be consulted. Since electrolyte abnormalities frequently occur with blood gas alterations, Table 5 shows these in the most common clinical disorders of blood gases. These are most helpful when a cardiorespiratory disorder complicates the picture.

In Section Four the common clinical disorders are discussed and illustrated with regard to pathophysiology, clinical picture, diagnosis and treatment.

Section Five deals with the essentials of fluid and electrolyte therapy.

Section Six presents case histories of 20 diagnostic and treatment problems with emphasis on the various combinations of diseases of electrolyte metabolism that one may encounter. For example Case 2 shows what happens to the electrolytes when a patient with pulmonary emphysema develops simultaneous renal failure and how the management must be altered.

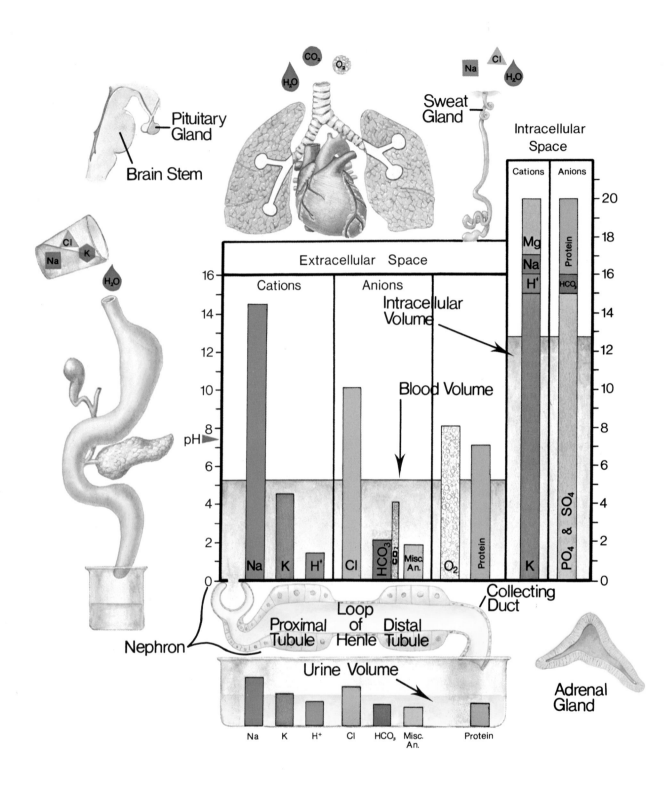

Explanation of the Basic Illustration

This illustration is a schematic representation of the body fluid and electrolytes, the compartments in which they reside, and the organs associated with their intake, absorption, transport, regulation and excretion. It would be impossible to illustrate in one drawing the exact amounts and relationship of all these components. Therefore, certain compromises have been made. Since the electrolyte composition of the extracellular fluid and plasma are very similar, these are superimposed upon each other. It should be remembered that the extracellular compartment is actually four times that of plasma (and includes the plasma compartment). Furthermore, the interstitial fluid (which fills three quarters of the extracellular compartment) contains very little protein compared to the plasma.

Plasma protein and P_{O_2} are represented in a neutral compartment even though protein does participate to some degree in the buffer system as anion. The most important role of protein is its osmotic effect on maintaining plasma volume. The oxygen content represented includes that carried by the red cells (very large) and that which is dissolved in the plasma (a small amount).

Hydrogen ion has been represented in plasma, interstitial fluid and intracellular fluid to a scale that suggests amounts far in excess of its actual concentration so that disorders of acid-base balance can be shown more clearly and better understood. The pH is also represented so that its reciprocal relationship with hydrogen ion can be depicted. Plasma calcium and magnesium purposely have been excluded because they contribute very little to an understanding of fluid and electrolyte disorders.

The intracellular compartment (normally two times the size of the extracellular space) has been considerably reduced in size so that it would fit into the drawing. The kidney is illustrated as a single nephron, since the function of all nephrons is similar. The electrolytes of the normal stool are not illustrated, since they contribute very little to an understanding of fluid and electrolyte disorders. Likewise, the amount of potassium lost from sweat normally is so minimal that it is not illustrated.

Summary of Normal Values Illustrated

Plasma Na—138-145 mEq./L.
Plasma K—3.5-4.5 mEq./L.
Plasma H^+—20-40 ng./L.
Plasma Cl—95-105 mEq./L.
Plasma HCO_3^-—21-25 mEq./L.
Blood P_{CO_2}—40-45 mm.
Miscellaneous anions—12 ± 4 mEq./L.

Blood P_{O_2}—75-100 mm.
Plasma protein—6-8 gm./100 ml.
Plasma pH—7.35-7.45
Intracellular magnesium—25-35 mEq./L.
Intracellular sodium—10-35 mEq./L
Intracellular hydrogen ion—40 ng./L.

Intracellular potassium—150 mEq./L.
Intracellular protein—40 mEq./L.
Intracellular HCO_3^-—10-20 mEq./L.
Intracellular phosphates and sulfates—150 mEq./L.
Intracellular fluid volume—40 percent of body weight

3

Section One
Normal Metabolism

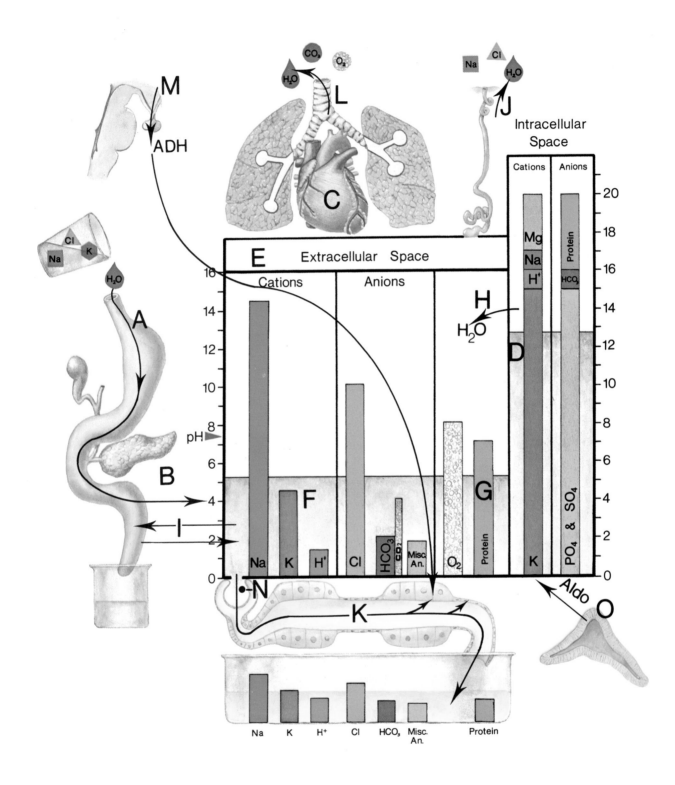

Water

Intake

The average normal adult ingests from 1,500 to 3,000 ml. of water a day via the gastrointestinal tract (A). This will be greatly increased when sensible (sweat) water loss increases during heavy labor. If there is no ingestion of water or other liquids the body can conserve water a great deal, but nevertheless at least 500 to 600 ml. is lost daily in the urine and 600 to 800 ml. through the skin and lungs in the form of insensible water loss.

Absorption

Water is thought to be absorbed from the intestinal mucosa (B) through aqueous-filled channels or pores in response to osmotic pressure differences between the plasma and intestinal contents.[14] At any one time 1.4 to 1.6 percent of body water lies in the gastrointestinal tract with electrolytes and food. This fluid is isosmotic with plasma except for saliva which is hypotonic.

Transport and Distribution

Water is transported to the tissues by the blood and lymphatics under the power of the heart (C) and the skeletal muscles. The total body water is between 50 and 70 percent of body weight depending on the amount of fatty tissue. In thin persons the total body water is closer to 70 percent while in obese people it is closer to 50 percent. The total body water of a 70-Kg. man of average build is 42 liters. Of the total body water approximately 55 percent (40 percent of body weight) is in the intracellular space (D), 16 percent (20 percent of body weight) is in the extracellular space (E) and 7.5 percent is in the plasma (F). Another 15 percent is in bone, cartilage and connective tissue. Thus the average 70-Kg. male has 30.8 liters of water intracellularly and 11.2 liters in the extracellular space of which 3.5 liters is in the plasma (*see Fig. 1*). The distribution between plasma and extracellular fluid is maintained by plasma protein (G) drawing water into the circulation balanced by the hydrostatic pressure from the heart, driving water out of the plasma. A loss of plasma protein allows more plasma water to escape into the extracellular space, and a weak heart may create backward failure and increased hydrostatic pressure in the veins, driving water into the extracellular space. The volume of intracellular water is maintained primarily by intracellular protein. However, if plasma water is reduced for whatever reason, plasma protein will compete with intracellular protein for water and gradu-

ally draw some of the water out of the cells. This is one of the ways circulatory volume is maintained effectively.

Production

Water is produced in the body by the cellular catabolism of protein, fat and carbohydrate (H). Approximately 300 ml. is produced each day in this manner. When there is significant cell breakdown in addition (as in starvation) a certain amount of intracellular water is released also.

Secretion

Over 8 liters of water rich in electrolytes is secreted and reabsorbed in the gastrointestinal tract daily (I). This can increase to as much as 30 liters a day in disease states associated with vomiting or diarrhea where there are immense losses. The sweat glands (J) can secrete up to 24 liters of water a day (sensible water loss). On the other hand they may secrete virtually none when necessary.

Excretion

The average adult excretes between 600 and 1,600 ml. of water a day in the urine (K). With normal influence of the pituitary and adrenal glands, the normal kidney will adjust the output according to the intake. However the normal kidney cannot reduce the excretion below 500 ml. a day so that its capacity to conserve water is limited. In addition at least 600 to 800 ml. of water is invariably lost via the lungs (L) and skin by evaporation (insensible water loss). Assuming that 300 ml. of water is produced each day by catabolism, the normal adult must ingest or take intravenously at least 1,000 ml. of water a day to maintain water balance. In practice it is well to allow enough intake for at least 1,000 ml. of urine output, 300 ml. of sweat, 800 ml. of insensible water loss and subtract from this the 300 ml. produced by catabolism. Thus a minimum of 1,800 ml. of fluid should be ingested by the average normal healthy adult each day.

Regulation

Several regulatory mechanisms have been hinted at in the above discussion. Two mechanisms are most influential in maintaining the volume and concentration (tonicity) of the body fluids in a normal range in the healthy adult. These are thirst and the kidney under the influence of antidiuretic hormone and aldosterone.

Thirst is stimulated by hypertonicity of the extracellular fluid and a contracted intracellular volume. It is depressed by hypotonicity of the extracellular fluid and an expanded intracellular fluid volume. It has been conclusively shown in animal experiments that the administration of hypertonic saline intravenously will induce the alert animal to drink water.[2] In elderly people and in diseased states this stimulus of thirst may be impaired.

Kidney. The mechanism of renal control of the volume and tonicity of body fluids is fascinating.

Tonicity. If the plasma, and hence the glomerular filtrate (a protein-free plasma filtrate with the same electrolyte composition as plasma), is hypertonic, the osmoreceptors in the supraoptic nucleus are stimulated to release antidiuretic hormone (ADH) (M). This makes the distal and collecting tubules more permeable to water from the filtrate and thus it is absorbed, diluting the blood and concentrating the urine. If the plasma is hypotonic, then the secretion of ADH is inhibited, and the distal and collecting tubule reabsorb less water from the filtrate, concentrating the blood and diluting the urine.

Volume. If the blood and the extracellular fluid are low in volume, volume receptors, probably located in the juxtaglomerular apparatus (N), secrete renin which activates angiotensin (transformed to angiotensin II by the lungs) to stimulate the adrenal cortex to secrete aldosterone (O), and more sodium is reabsorbed from the filtrate in exchange for potassium and hydrogen ions. The resulting hypertonicity of the plasma will lead to ADH secretion and water retention, as described above. Hypovolemia also seems to be an important stimulus of ADH secretion.[8] Thus the volume is returned to normal. A large plasma volume will lead to suppression of aldosterone secretion in like manner, with a consequent decrease in tubular reabsorption of sodium. Intravascular and extracellular volume is adjusted by the intracellular water in many disease states. When there is water loss with resulting hypertonicity of extracellular fluid, water moves out of the cell. When there is excess extracellular water and hypotonicity, the reverse occurs.

Pathophysiology of Deficits or Excesses. A *deficit* in body water may result from reduced ingestion (dehydration), increased excretion by the kidney either from renal disease or secondary to ADH deficiency, or from excretion via an abnormal pathway (vomiting, or diarrhea, excessive sweating or excessive respiration).

An *excess* in body water may result from increased ingestion or intravenous administration, decreased excretion by a diseased kidney or a kidney stimulated by excess ADH or inadequate transport of water to the kidney (as in shock or congestive heart failure).

Sodium

Intake

Sodium enters the body via the gastrointestinal tract (A) by ingestion with foodstuffs. The average normal adult ingests from 69 to 208 mEq. of sodium each day.

Absorption

Sodium is absorbed from the small intestine (B) by an as yet unknown active diffusion process.

Transport

Once absorbed, sodium is transported by the blood where its concentration is normally 135 to 145 mEq./L. The power for its transport is the heart (C) and skeletal muscle.

Production

Sodium is not produced by the body, but the small amount of sodium that exists intracellularly (D) may be released into the blood when there is severe hyponatremia or acidosis (when it is exchanged for hydrogen ion).

Storage

Forty percent of the body sodium exists in the blood and extracellular fluid. The rest is intracellular (35 mEq./L.) and in bone and connective tissue. Much of the sodium in bone is exchangeable so that, combined with extracellular sodium, 70 percent is exchangeable. Total body sodium is 58 mEq. per Kg. so that a 70-Kg. male has approximately 4,000 mEq. of sodium and 2,800 mEq. (70 percent) of this is in the blood, extracellular fluid, or easily displaced from bone and connective tissue in time of need.

Secretion

Sodium is secreted in sweat (45 mEq./L.) (E), the gastric juice (20-100 mEq./L.) (F), and the pancreatic fluid, bile and small intestines (80-150 mEq./L.) (G). Most of that which is secreted into the gastrointestinal tract is reabsorbed, so that only 10 mEq. or less pass into the stool each day. However, massive amounts of sodium may be lost in gastrointestinal diseases associated with vomiting or diarrhea. Sodium secreted in the sweat is not reabsorbed. Large amounts of sodium may be lost in this way under pathologic conditions.

Excretion

Sodium is excreted by the kidney (H) in amounts equal to that ingested minus what is lost in the sweat. The average adult will excrete 100 to 140 mEq. of sodium a day through the kidney in a cool environment. The body can conserve sodium so that urine output on a salt-free diet may drop to 10 mEq. a day. It is understandable that it should, since sodium is the major ion responsible for maintaining blood volume and hence circulation. The mechanisms of excretion of body sodium are intimately related to its regulation so these will be discussed together.

Regulation

The kidney regulates sodium excretion according to body needs primarily under the influence of the renin-angiotensin-aldosterone system (I). Unlike potassium "regulation," sodium regulation is not accomplished by secretion of sodium. Sodium passes through the glomerulus at a concentration of 142 mEq./L. (approximately). In the proximal tubule (J) 60 to 70 percent of this is absorbed by an osmotic gradient, a chemical and electrical gradient. The osmotic gradient is the pull of the colloid (protein) in the peritubular capillaries. The chemical gradient is probably related to the exchange of sodium for hydrogen ion to form bicarbonate. The electrical gradient operates like a sodium pump and sodium is absorbed with chloride in this manner. In the ascending limb of Henle (K) 20 to 25 percent more sodium is absorbed with chloride. This is a hypertonic reabsorption.[2] It is in the distal tubule (L) that the major influence of aldosterone is brought to bear (although some studies suggest an additional effect on the loop of Henle[3]). In the distal tubule sodium is reabsorbed in exchange for hydrogen ion or potassium depending on body needs. The hydrogen ion competes with potassium for the exchange with sodium so that if there is acidosis or hypokalemia more hydrogen ion will be exchanged for sodium, whereas if there is alkalosis or hyperkalemia more potassium ion will be exchanged for sodium.

Although a low concentration of sodium may act directly on the adrenal cortex to secrete aldosterone, the primary stimulus for aldosterone secretion comes from hypovolemia. A low blood volume stimulates volume receptors in the juxtaglomerular apparatus to secrete renin. This promotes the conversion of angiotensinogen to angiotensin I which is subsequently converted to angiotensin II by the lungs.

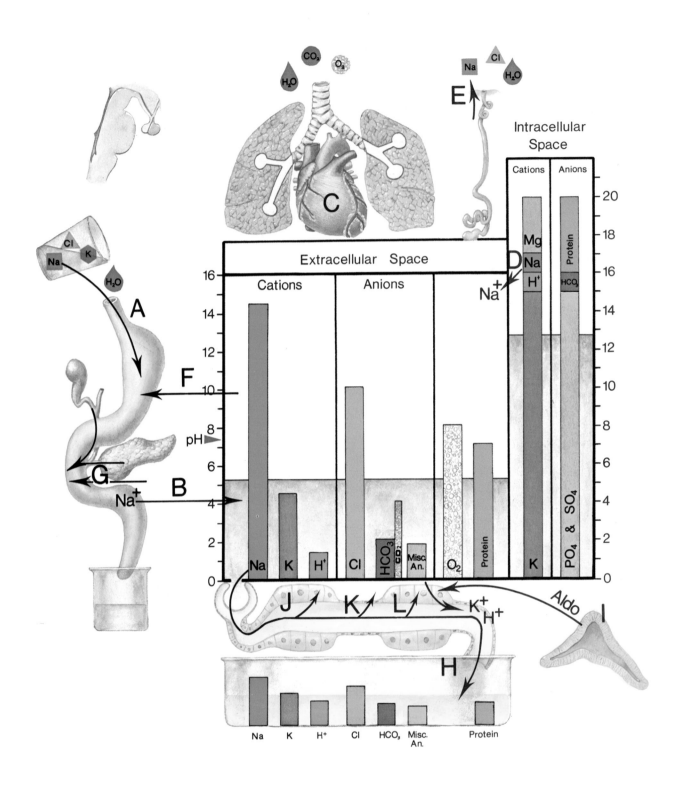

Angiotensin II stimulates the adrenal cortex to release aldosterone. Aldosterone enhances the distal tubular reabsorption of sodium in exchange for potassium and hydrogen ions. The resulting hypernatremia is only momentary of course because it stimulates osmoreceptors in the supraoptic nucleus to release ADH and this acts on the distal tubule and collecting ducts to retain water.

Just as a low blood volume will lead to a stimulation of the above events, a high blood volume will lead to a suppression of aldosterone and ADH with a greater loss of sodium and water in the urine. It should be pointed out that in addition to aldosterone other factors such as arterial pressure, renal vascular resistance and compositional changes of plasma may influence sodium reabsorption.[2]

Pathophysiology of Deficits and Excesses

Hyponatremia may result from decreased intake, decreased absorption (malabsorption syndrome), increased secretion (pathologic diaphoresis and secretory diarrhea), increased output (diuretics), retention of water out of proportion to salt (inappropriate ADH syndrome) and poor transport of water and salt to the kidney for excretion (congestive heart failure). A disturbance of regulation (adrenal insufficiency) may also cause hyponatremia. Hyperglycemia and hyperlipidemia reduce the laboratory value for sodium, but do not cause an actual reduction in serum sodium.

Hypernatremia rarely results from increased intake of salt, but can result from either decreased intake of water (dehydration), increased excretion of water (diabetes insipidus, etc.) or a disorder of regulation (aldosteronism).

When sodium is retained in hypertension, renal failure and congestive heart failure, water is usually retained with it so that the concentration of sodium is usually low or within normal limits.

See Table 3 for a more detailed list of the causes of hyponatremia and hypernatremia.

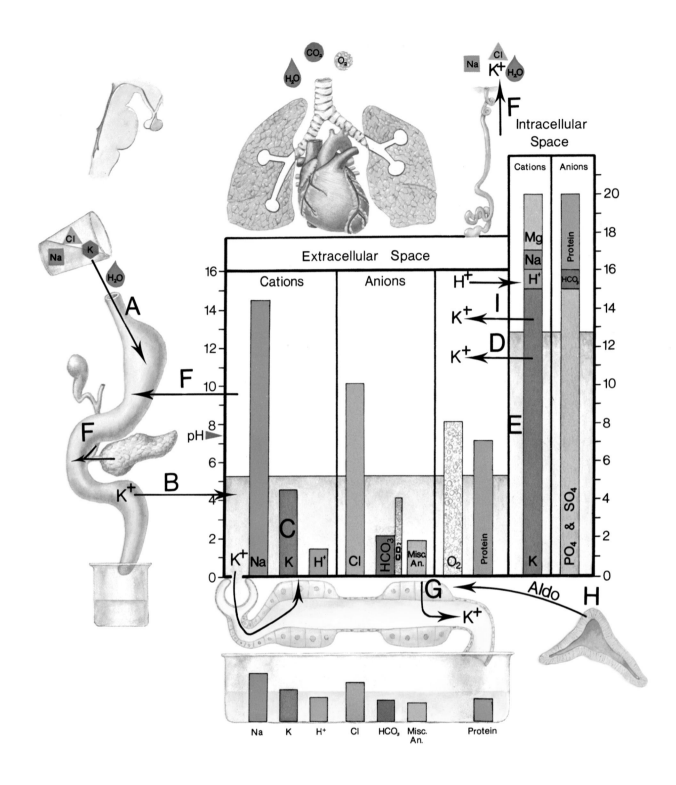

Potassium

Intake

Potassium enters the body by ingestion into the gastrointestinal tract (A). The average adult ingests from 50 to 120 mEq. a day with food and drink. Fruits such as oranges, bananas and prunes contain large amounts of potassium.

Absorption

Potassium is absorbed in the small intestines (B) by an as yet unknown active diffusion process. Only about 5 to 10 mEq. of intake passes into the stool, except when there is diarrhea (page 101).

Transport

Potassium is transported in the blood and lymphatics under the force of the heart and the skeletal muscles. The normal concentration varies between 3.8 and 5 mEq./L. in both blood and extracellular fluid (C).

Production

Potassium is not produced in the body, but it may be released from the cells (D) when the body relies on cell catabolism for energy.

Storage

Most of the body potassium is in the intracellular fluid (E) where its concentration is 150 to 160 mEq/L. There is approximately 3,600 mEq. of potassium in a 70/Kg. healthy male.

Secretion

Potassium is secreted in sweat (5 mEq./L.), gastric juice (5-25 mEq/L.), pancreatic juice (3-10 mEq./L.), bile (3-12 mEq./L.) and fluids of the small intestine (2-10 mEq./L.) (F). These secretions are a potential source of great losses in gastrointestinal diseases.

Excretion

Ninety percent of ingested potassium is excreted by the kidney, the rest is lost through the sweat and the stool. All the potassium filtered by the glomerulus is reabsorbed, but nevertheless 60 to 90 mEq. are secreted by the distal tubule (G) each day in exchange for sodium. Although the body can conserve sodium, when there is lack of potassium intake it continues to excrete 50 mEq. of potassium daily long after intake has ceased.

Regulation

Mineralocorticoids (aldosterone, etc.) increase the secretion of potassium in exchange for sodium (H). When there is acidosis, potassium moves out of the cell in exchange for hydrogen ions (I) and more hydrogen ions and less potassium ions are exchanged for sodium in the distal tubule. Thus serum potassium may rise. In alkalosis the reverse occurs. As glucose enters the cell it takes potassium with it. This process may be used to lower serum potassium.

Pathophysiology of Deficits and Excesses

Hypokalemia may result from decreased intake, decreased absorption, increased secretion (as in diarrhea and vomiting), increased excretion (diuretics) or a disturbance in regulation (aldosteronism).

Hyperkalemia usually results from decreased excretion (renal failure) but may result from disorders of regulation (acidosis, aldosterone antagonists) and increased intravenous administration.

See Table 3 for a more detailed list of the causes of hypokalemia and hyperkalemia.

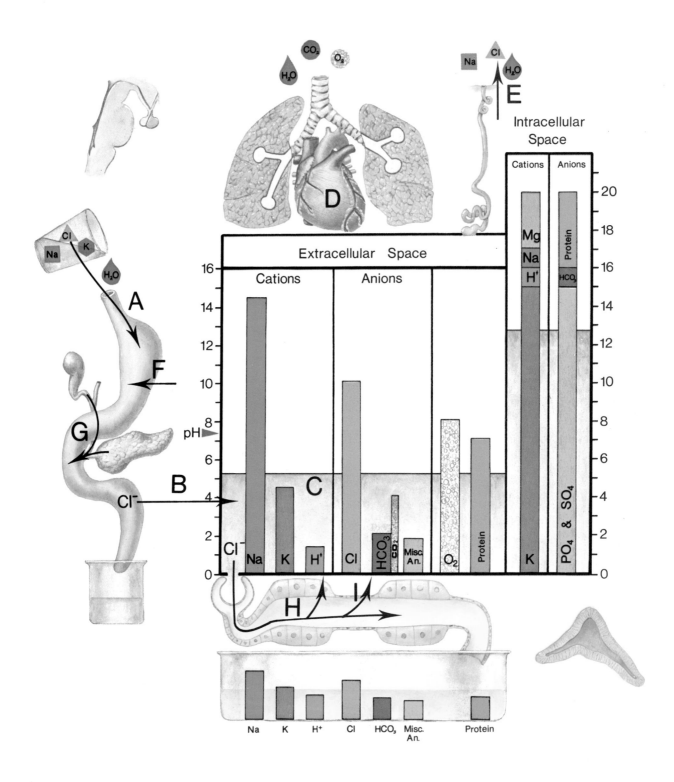

Chloride

With the exception of a few subtleties, the normal metabolism of chloride closely parallels that of sodium.

Intake

The average normal adult ingests via the gastrointestinal tract (A) 69 to 208 mEq. of chloride in food and drink, usually as the sodium or potassium salt. The minimum daily requirement is 75 mEq.

Absorption

Chloride is absorbed in the small intestine (B) along with sodium and potassium and other salts by an as yet unknown active diffusion process.

Transport

Chloride, like sodium, is transported in the blood (C) and lymphatics under the force of the heart (D) and the skeletal muscles. Chloride is the principal anion of the blood and the extracellular fluid. Normal blood levels are 100 ± 8 mEq./L.[4]

Secretion

Chloride is secreted in sweat (E) with sodium (45 mEq./L.), in gastric juice (F) with hydrogen ions (90-155 mEq./L.), and in bile, pancreatic and intestinal fluids (G) with sodium (approximately 100 mEq./L.).

Excretion

It is in the renal tubules (H) that sodium and chloride often part ways. Depending on the body's need for sodium bicarbonate, more or less chloride is dumped in the urine as the ammonium salt to eliminate hydrogen ions in exchange for sodium. Thus the tubule secretes NH_3 and H^+ into the tubular lumen and reabsorbs sodium along with the bicarbonate formed in the tubular cell. The following diagram summarizes this event:

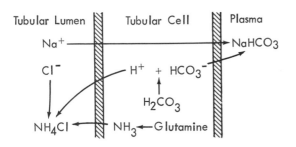

This reaction may occur anywhere along the nephron, but primarily in the proximal tubule. Chloride is absorbed almost exclusively with sodium in the ascending loop of Henle (I). However, it may be absorbed anywhere along the nephron.

Regulation

Regulation of the chloride level in the blood is passively related to the sodium level. When serum sodium increases, chloride usually increases. However, chloride blood levels are related inversely to blood levels of bicarbonate because, as stated above, chloride will be sacrificed in the urine to produce more bicarbonate. Bicarbonate production is under the influence of aldosterone so that this hormone indirectly influences chloride levels.

Pathophysiology of Deficits and Excesses

Hypochloremia is seen where there is *increased secretion* and loss of gastric juice (pyloric obstruction, etc.), *increased* renal *excretion* (mercurial diuretics, etc.), disorders of *regulation* (aldosteronism), *hemodilution* (e.g., dilutional hyponatremia), *actual hyponatremia* (pathologic diaphoresis) and acidotic states where increased production of bicarbonate is necessary (pulmonary emphysema, etc.).

Hyperchloremia results when there is excessive *intake* or administration of salt, decreased production of bicarbonate to compensate for a respiratory alkalosis, *decreased excretion* by a kidney unable to make bicarbonate (renal tubular acidosis, etc.), dehydration, and excessive *reabsorption* from the gastrointestinal tract (uretero-ileostomies). For a more detailed list of causes of hypochloremia and hyperchloremia see Table 3.

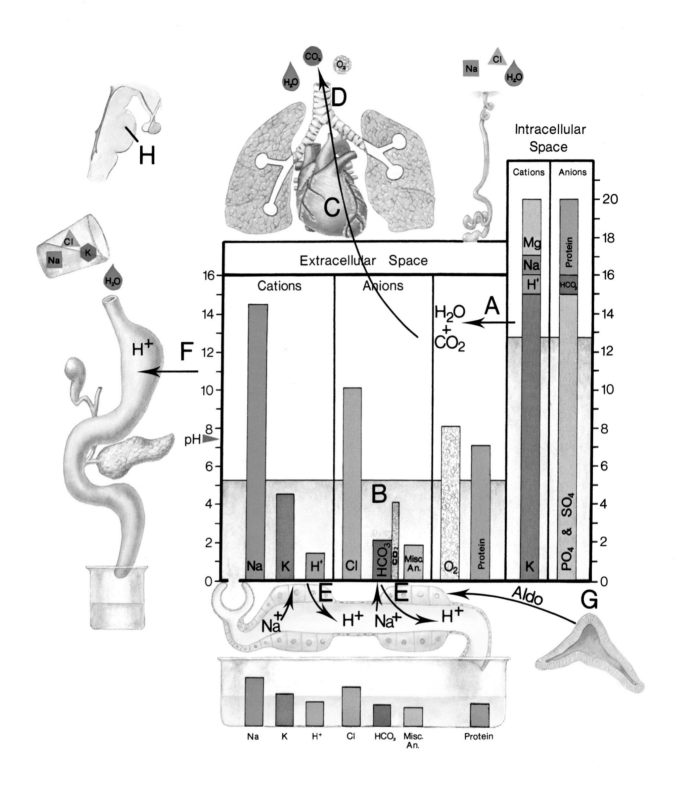

Hydrogen Ion, Carbon Dioxide and Bicarbonate

Since the metabolism of these three are intimately related in health and disease they will be discussed together.

Intake and Absorption

The intake or ingestion and absorption of hydrogen ion, carbon dioxide and bicarbonate through the lungs and gastrointestinal tract is negligible under normal circumstances. Patients with chronic peptic ulcer disease may develop a milk-alkali syndrome (page 81) from ingestion of too much sodium bicarbonate.

Production

Hydrogen ion, carbon dioxide and bicarbonate basically originate in one source: the catabolism of carbohydrate, fat and protein by the cells to form water and carbon dioxide (A). A small amount of hydrogen ion originates from the oxidation of sulfur-containing amino acids to sulfuric acids, the oxidation of phosphoproteins to phosphoric acid and a small amount of fat and carbohydrate that is incompletely oxidized to organic acids.[2] Approximately 60 to 70 mEq. of these acids are generated each day.

The cells release 20,000 mEq. of carbon dioxide each day. In order to maintain acid-base equilibrium, almost all of this is transported to the lungs and exhaled. A small amount of this remains dissolved in the blood as "free carbon dioxide" or attached to hemoglobin. This value can be determined by measuring the arterial P_{CO_2}. This is normally 40 ± 2 mm. Hg. The carbon dioxide then combines with water to form carbonic acid as follows:

$$(1) \quad CO_2 + H_2O \longrightarrow H_2CO_3$$

The H_2CO_3 dissociates to release H^+ as follows:

$$(2) \quad H_2CO_3 \longrightarrow H^+ + HCO_3^-$$

Actually at any one time only $1/800$ of the free carbon dioxide is in the form of carbonic acid (1.1-1.3 mEq./L.) and only a small amount of this is dissociated into H^+ and HCO_3^-. The hydrogen ion concentration of arterial blood is between $1/10^7$ and $1/10^8$ mEq./L.[4] But the potential to form more carbonic acid (and thus more H^+) from carbon dioxide is there in alkalotic states, particularly when respirations are slowed to decrease the excretion of carbon dioxide. However, since the body is continuously forming acid during metabolism the potential to combat acidosis is much greater. This is where bicarbonate comes in.

The formation of bicarbonate means simply taking the dissolved carbon dioxide and consequent carbonic acid one step further. The kidney is primarily responsible for this job, since it is richly supplied with carbonic anhydrase.[5] Equations (1) and (2) above are promoted as follows:

$$CO_2 + H_2O \xrightarrow{\;CA\;} H_2CO_3 \longrightarrow H^+ + HCO_3^- \quad (3)$$

As sodium flows through the tubular lumen it is "switched" for hydrogen ion and reabsorbed as bicarbonate by three different mechanisms.[7]

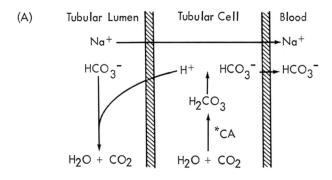

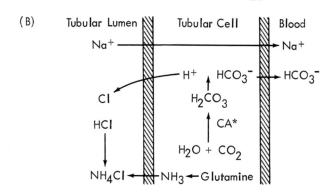

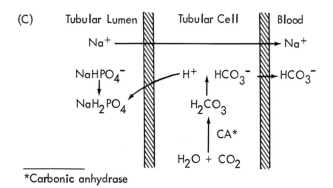

*Carbonic anhydrase

A large amount of sodium bicarbonate is formed in this manner. At the normal pH of the body there is 20 times more bicarbonate than carbonic acid as demonstrated by the Henderson-Hasselbalch equation.

$$pH = pK + \log \frac{[HCO_3^-]}{[H_2CO_3]} \qquad (4)$$

If pH is 7.4 (normal) and pK is 6.1

$$\text{then } \frac{[HCO_3^-]}{[H_2CO_3]} = \frac{20}{1} \qquad (5)$$

Since $NaHCO_3$ represents almost all of the HCO_3^- and P_{CO_2} forms the carbonic acid it is easier to understand the above if it is changed to:

$$\frac{[NaHCO_3]}{[CO_2]} = \frac{20}{1}$$

Some bicarbonate is formed in other areas of the body where carbonic anhydrase activity exists (see below).

Since clinical laboratories report the plasma bicarbonate either as total CO_2 (CO_2 content) or HCO_3^- these two designations are used interchangeably. Actually the total CO_2 of plasma is the HCO_3^- plus 1.1 to 1.3 milliequivalents of H_2CO_3.

Transport

Hydrogen ion, carbon dioxide and bicarbonate are transported by the blood (B) under the force of the heart (C) and skeletal muscle. The hydrogen ion concentration of arterial blood is between $^1/_{10}{}^7$ and $^1/_{10}{}^8$ mEq./L. but it appears to be more in the illustration for the sake of clarity. The normal arterial carbon dioxide is 40 ± 2 mm. Hg. Bicarbonate ranges between 21 and 25 mEq./L. The total carbon dioxide content of plasma ranges between 22 and 27 mEq./L.

Excretion

Most of the 20,000 mEq. of carbon dioxide formed each day is eliminated by the lungs (D) but some is used by the kidney to form bicarbonate (as described above). It follows that most of the hydrogen ion is eliminated by the conversion of carbonic acid to CO_2 and water ($H^+ + HCO_3^- \longrightarrow H_2O + CO_2$). However some is eliminated by secretion through the renal tubules (E) in exchange for sodium when bicarbonate is being formed. About 4,200 mEq. of hydrogen ion are excreted daily in this fashion. Finally a small amount of hydrogen ion (60-70 mEq.) is excreted by the kidney with miscellaneous anions (phosphates, sulfates and ketones, etc.). Almost all of the bicarbonate reaching the kidney in the normal individual is reabsorbed. However, when there is chronic alkali administration as much as 1,200 mEq. of bicarbonate can be excreted daily in the urine. The

"alkaline tide" of bicarbonate formed in the production of hydrochloric acid by the stomach (see below) is also excreted by the kidney following meals.

Secretion

The hydrogen ion "secreted" by the kidney has already been discussed. There is also hydrogen ion secretion by the stomach (F) in the formation of hydrochloric acid. One proposed mechanism for this is as follows:

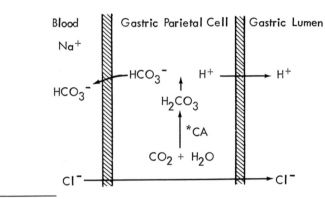

*Carbonic anhydrase

The maximal hydrogen ion concentration of this secretion is about 0.16 N, or a 0.16 N solution of hydrochloric acid.[6]

Bicarbonate is secreted by the bile, pancreas and intestines to aid the digestive enzymes in these fluids.

Regulation

Regulation of hydrogen ion, carbon dioxide and bicarbonate is performed primarily by the lungs (D) and kidneys (E) under the influence of the adrenal cortex (G) and the respiratory centers in the brain stem (H).

Were it not for these remarkable homeostatic mechanisms of the lung and kidney, the blood would quickly become acid.[7]

In the first place, the average diet contains substances with acid end-products (ammonium salts, sulfur-containing amino acids, phosphoric acid compounds). Furthermore, carbon dioxide is constantly being poured into the blood as the end-product of cellular metabolism of carbohydrates and fats. To a lesser degree, ketoacids are being produced in fat metabolism. All these substances are buffered by the bicarbonate, phosphate and other buffer systems of the blood so that the blood pH does not change radically from the normal range of 7.35 to 7.45. These buffers and particularly the bicarbonate must be maintained.

Lung. When carbon dioxide is released by the cells or by the buffering of ingested acids it stimulates the respiratory center to increase respirations so that it can be excreted by the lungs. When an alkaline solution (sodium bicarbonate) is ingested or injected into the blood, the respiratory center is depressed so that less carbon dioxide is given off and more carbonic acid is maintained in the blood to equalize the sodium bicarbonate and keep the pH between 7.35 and 7.45.

Kidney. When an acid is poured into the blood it is buffered by the sodium bicarbonate in the following manner:

$$H^+ A^- + NaHCO_3 \longrightarrow NaA + H_2CO_3$$

The phosphate buffer system acts in a similar manner:

$$H^+ A^- + Na_2HPO_4 \longrightarrow NaA + NaH_2PO_4$$

Other buffer systems react in a similar manner. These buffers must be restored by the kidneys. It does this in three ways: (1) by reabsorbing almost all the sodium bicarbonate from the glomerular filtrate, (2) by acidifying urinary buffer salts such as disodium phosphate, and (3) by excreting hydrogen ion as the ammonium salt of strong acids (HCl, etc.). All three mechanisms are based on one fundamental process. This is the tubular secretion of hydrogen ion in exchange for sodium in the tubular urine. A read-ily available source of hydrogen ion is provided by the conversion of water and carbon dioxide to carbonic acid under the influence of carbonic anhydrase (as described above) in the tubular cell. The hydrogen ion of the carbonic acid is then exchanged for the sodium of sodium bicarbonate, sodium diphosphate and other salts (sodium chloride) of the glomerular filtrate in the following manner:

$$NaHCO_3 \xrightarrow{H^+} H_2CO_3 + Na^+$$

$$Na_2HPO_4 \xrightarrow{H^+} NaH_2PO_4 + Na^+$$

$$NaCl \xrightarrow[NH_3]{H^+} NH_4Cl + Na^+$$

(Ammonium is added by the tubular cells in the last equation.) The sodium released by these mechanisms combines with the bicarbonate of the tubular cell and enters the blood as sodium bicarbonate. The secretion of hydrogen ion in exchange for sodium can be augmented by aldosterone from the adrenal cortex (G).

When an alkaline substance (sodium bicarbonate) is poured into the blood, all the above mechanisms can be depressed so that sodium bicarbonate and other buffer salts (sodium diphosphate) are excreted in the urine.

To summarize these compensatory mechanisms of the lung and kidney one can utilize the "tail" of the Henderson-Hasselbalch equation to show what happens:

(1) CO_2 retention (respiratory acidosis)

$$\underset{\text{(Normal)}}{\frac{20\ NaHCO_3}{1\ CO_2}} + 2\ CO_2 \longrightarrow \underset{\text{(Uncompensated)}}{\frac{20\ NaHCO_3}{3\ CO_2}} + \underset{\substack{\text{(produced by} \\ \text{kidney)}}}{40\ NaHCO_3} \longrightarrow \underset{\text{(Compensated)}}{\frac{60\ NaHCO_3}{3\ CO_2}} = \frac{20}{1}$$

(2) CO_2 excretion increased (respiratory alkalosis)

$$\underset{\text{(Normal)}}{\frac{20\ NaHCO_3}{1\ CO_2}} - 0.5\ CO_2 \longrightarrow \underset{\text{(Uncompensated)}}{\frac{20\ NaHCO_3}{0.5\ CO_2}} - \underset{\substack{\text{(excreted by} \\ \text{kidney)}}}{10\ NaHCO_3} \longrightarrow \underset{\text{(Compensated)}}{\frac{10 NaHCO_3}{0.5\ CO_2}} = \frac{20}{1}$$

(3) Bicarbonate used up or lost (metabolic acidosis)

$$\underset{\text{(Normal)}}{\frac{20\ NaHCO_3}{1\ CO_2}} - 10\ NaHCO_3 \longrightarrow \underset{\text{(Uncompensated)}}{\frac{10\ NaHCO_3}{1\ CO_2}} - \underset{\substack{\text{(excreted by} \\ \text{hyperventilation)}}}{0.5\ CO_2} \longrightarrow \underset{\text{(Compensated)}}{\frac{10\ NaHCO_3}{0.5\ CO_2}} = \frac{20}{1}$$

(4) Bicarbonate excess (metabolic alkalosis)

$$\underset{\text{(Normal)}}{\frac{20\ NaHCO_3}{1\ CO_2}} + 20\ NaHCO_3 \longrightarrow \underset{\text{(Uncompensated)}}{\frac{40\ NaHCO_3}{1\ CO_2}} + \underset{\substack{\text{(retained by} \\ \text{hypoventilation)}}}{1\ CO_2} \longrightarrow \underset{\text{(Compensated)}}{\frac{40\ NaHCO_3}{2\ CO_2}} = \frac{20}{1}$$

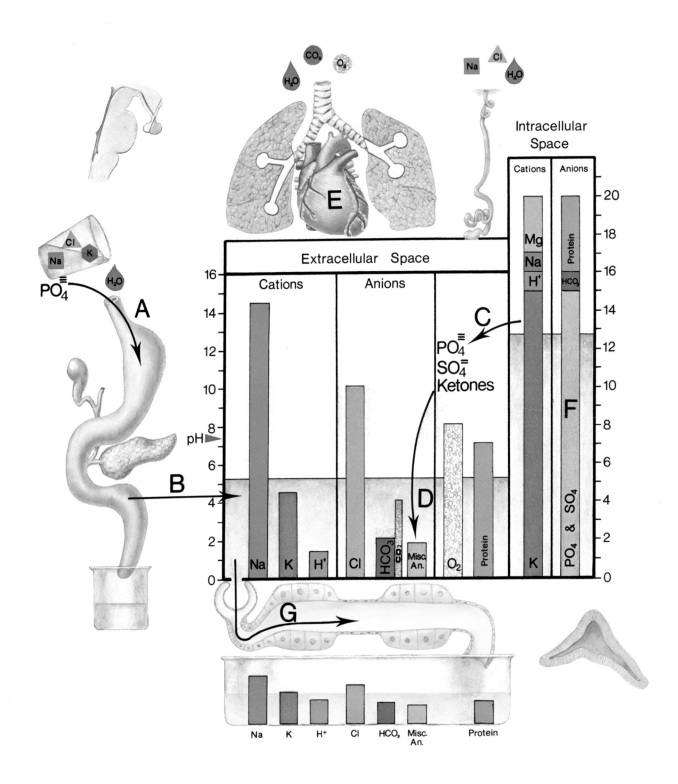

Thus a respiratory acidosis is compensated for by kidney formation, or "retention" of sodium bicarbonate; a respiratory alkalosis is compensated for by kidney excretion of sodium bicarbonate; a metabolic acidosis is compensated for by lung hyperventilation of carbon dioxide and a metabolic alkalosis is compensated for by lung hypoventilation of carbon dioxide.

Pathophysiology of Deficits and Excesses

Hydrogen ion deficits (alkalosis) result from an increased excretion of carbon dioxide (hyperventilation syndrome, salicylate intoxication) or increased excretion of acid (vomiting) or an increased ingestion of alkali (milk-alkali syndrome) or an increased formation of bicarbonate (aldosteronism).

Hydrogen ion excess (acidosis) results from decreased excretion of carbon dioxide (pulmonary emphysema), increased excretion of bicarbonate (diarrhea) or increased production of acid by the body (diabetic ketoacidosis) or decreased excretion of acids by the body (acute renal failure) and decreased production of bicarbonate (renal tubular acidosis).

Carbon dioxide deficits result from increased excretion of carbon dioxide (salicylate intoxication) and as compensation for a metabolic acidosis.

Carbon dioxide excesses result from decreased excretion of carbon dioxide (pulmonary emphysema) and as compensation for a metabolic alkalosis.

Bicarbonate deficits result from increased ingestion of acids, decreased production by the kidney (renal tubular acidosis), increased utilization in buffering acids formed by the body (diabetic ketoacidosis), or increased excretion (diarrhea).

Bicarbonate excesses result from increased ingestion of alkaline solutions (milk-alkali syndrome), increased excretion of acid (vomiting), or increased production (aldosteronism).

For a more complete list of causes of the above alterations see Table 3.

Miscellaneous Anions

Definition

The miscellaneous anions of the body include sulfate, phosphate, ketones and a small amount of lactic acid. Some authors[4] include proteinate anions in this fraction, but this has already been designated as a separate entity in the illustration. The miscellaneous anions constitute the anion gap and are usually 12 ± 4 mEq./L. in plasma when matched with the cations exclusive of calcium and magnesium.

Intake

Phosphates are ingested as sodium, calcium and other salts via the gastrointestinal tract (A). Some phosphates and most of the other miscellaneous anions are ingested as protein and fat compounds so that they are not released from these until they are metabolized.

Absorption

Phosphates are absorbed in both the stomach and small intestine (B).

Production

Phosphates, sulfates and a small amount of ketones and lactic acid are released in the normal catabolism of ingested protein and fat. They may also be released in cell breakdown (C).

Transport

The miscellaneous anions are transported by the blood (D) under the force of the heart (E) and skeletal muscles. Their blood level is 12 ± 4 mEq./L.

Storage

Miscellaneous anions, particularly phosphates and sulfates, constitute the major intracellular anions (F). Phosphates and sulfates are also stored in bone with calcium and sodium. Thus they are important buffers both in and out of the cells.

Excretion

All the miscellaneous anions pass through the glomeruli (G). Only phosphates are reabsorbed accordingly to body needs. Phosphates can exchange sodium for hydrogen ions and thus help regenerate bicarbonate.

Regulation

The rate of cell breakdown has some effect on miscellaneous anions, but only indirectly. Phosphate reabsorption in the renal tubules is inhibited by parathyroid hormone. Since serum calcium is inversely related to serum phosphates, this effect allows more calcium to be mobilized from bone.

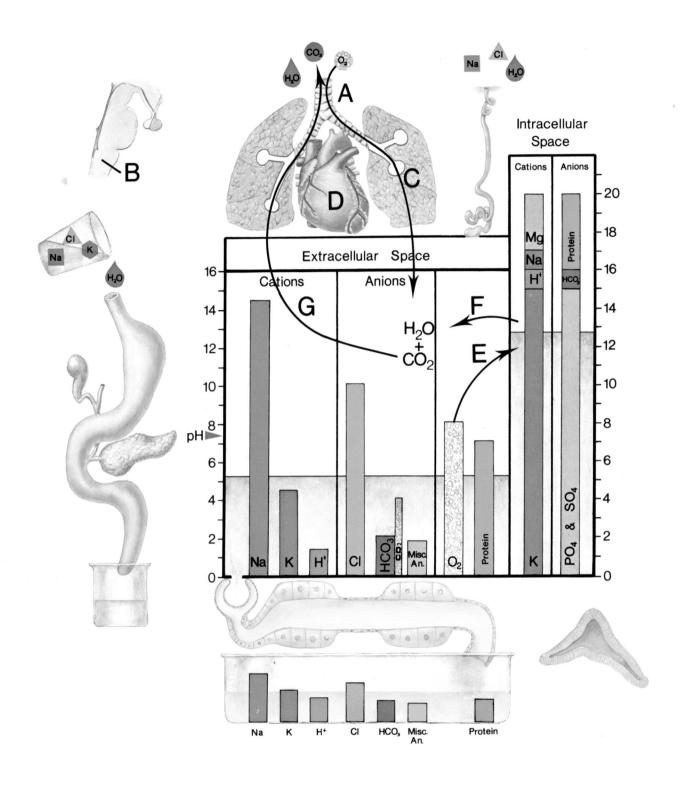

Intracellular Space

Cations   Anions

Extracellular Space

Cations   Anions

pH

H_2O + CO_2

Pathophysiology of Deficits and Excesses

Hypophosphatemia may occur when there is decreased intake or absorption, increased excretion (as in Fanconi syndrome) or a disorder of regulation (hyperparathyroidism).

Combined increases of phosphates and sulfates occur primarily with decreased excretion (renal failure), but increased phosphate may also occur with disturbed regulation (hypoparathyroidism).

Ketonemia occurs in disorders of increased fat breakdown (diabetes mellitus, starvation). *Lactic acidemia* occurs when there is increased production or decreased conversion of lactic acid to pyruvate. See Table 3 for a more detailed list of causes of the above deficits and excesses.

Oxygen

Intake

Oxygen intake may be considered the most important part of ventilation. Oxygen enters the body through the nose or mouth and travels through the pharynx, larynx, trachea, bronchi, bronchioles, and alveolar ducts (A) to the alveoli (C), where it may be absorbed into the blood stream. Because very little oxygen can be absorbed in the respiratory passages (the larynx, trachea, etc.), these are called "the anatomic dead air spaces" (in extent, approximately 150 ml.).

The amount of oxygen that might reach the alveoli by simple diffusion down the air passages would be inadequate to sustain life. Thus nature has developed an "air pump" made up of the thoracic cage, the diaphragm, and the elastic tissue in the walls of the lungs. Just as the heart pumps blood through the circulatory system, so this mechanism pumps air in and out of the lungs under the influence of the respiratory centers in the brain stem (B). During *inspiration* the external intercostal muscles contract, pulling the ribs upward and increasing the volume of the thorax. At the same time the diaphragmatic muscles may contract, lowering the level of the diaphragm and increasing the volume of the thorax. In this fashion air is drawn into the lungs.

In *expiration* the recoil ("resistance") of the elastic tissues of the lungs and thorax presses air out of the lungs. This elastic resistance is called "compliance" and may be measured. Ordinarily, this is a passive process. However, active expiration may be accomplished by contraction of the abdominal muscles, forcing the diaphragm up against the lungs and expressing more air.

Thus the intake of oxygen depends on patent respiratory passages, good neuromuscular function, a mobile and elastic thoracic cage, and elastic lungs; the rate and depth of respirations are determined by an intact respiratory center in the brain stem. Intake also depends on how much air the lungs can hold (total lung capacity). Each of these capacities can be measured.

Absorption

Oxygen is absorbed in the alveoli (C), which under normal conditions are richly supplied with capillaries. Collectively, the alveoli constitute an absorbing surface of 50 to 100 sq. m. To get to the blood, the oxygen molecules must diffuse across a surface film (covering the alveolar membrane), the alveolar membrane, the interstitial fluid, and a capillary membrane. Any of these layers may be thickened in disease states and prevent or decrease the absorption of oxygen.

From the above it is evident that oxygen absorption may be influenced by the total surface area of the alveoli and the character of the alveolar-capillary membranes. It is also influenced by the partial pressure of oxygen in the alveolar air (and thus the atmosphere). Normally, this must be greater than the partial pressure of oxygen in pulmonary capillary blood.

Oxygen absorption is also influenced by the partial pressure of carbon dioxide in the alveolar air and blood. High concentrations of carbon dioxide in the blood tend to inhibit the uptake of oxygen. Low concentrations of carbon dioxide in the blood have a reverse effect.

Furthermore, for adequate absorption to take place, the alveoli must be well ventilated and well supplied with pulmonary capillary blood. One is no good without the other. If an alveolus is well ventilated, but has no functioning capillaries (as in a pulmonary embolus), there will be no absorption of oxygen. Likewise, if an alveolus is well supplied with functioning capillaries, but is inadequately ventilated (as in atelectasis), there will be no oxygen absorption.

When some alveoli are better ventilated than others, there is said to be an uneven distribution of inspired gas. Such a situation occurs in many pulmonary diseases. The tests that have been developed to measure this will be discussed below. The distribution of pulmonary capillary blood flow may also be uneven. Direct measurement of this is more difficult. It should be emphasized that overall alveolar ventilation and pulmonary capillary blood flow may be adequate, and yet there may be anoxemia and carbon dioxide retention if alveoli that are ventilated are not well perfused, and if those that are well perfused are not well ventilated.

Transport

Following absorption, oxygen is carried to the tissues by the blood in the circulatory system under the force of the heart (D). The rate and stroke volume of the heart are adjusted to meet the oxygen needs of the body. Most of the oxygen is carried by the hemoglobin of the red cells. One gram of hemoglobin can hold 1.34 ml. of oxygen. The normal partial pressure of oxygen (PO_2) of arterial blood varies between 75 and 100 mm. depending on age.

Thus, transport of oxygen will be inadequate if there is inadequate hemoglobin (as in anemia); if some of the hemoglobin is altered in such a way that it cannot carry oxygen (as in methemoglobinemia); or if the heart is not capable of pumping the blood to the tissues (as in heart failure). Finally, some tissues may not receive adequate oxygen when blood is temporarily shunted to more vital tissues (shock).

Utilization

Oxygen is utilized by the tissues (E) in the aerobic catabolism of carbohydrate, fat, and protein, with the formation of carbon dioxide (F), water, and other waste products. Adequate utilization depends on many cellular enzymes.

Excretion

Oxygen, following its utilization, is excreted in the form of carbon dioxide and water. Water may be excreted in a variety of ways (kidney, lungs, skin, etc.). Although some carbon dioxide is excreted as bicarbonate in the urine, most of the carbon dioxide is excreted by way of the lungs (G).

Carbon dioxide is transported to the lungs in the blood as free carbon dioxide, bicarbonate, in combination with plasma proteins, or as carboxyhemoglobin. In the lungs it diffuses from the blood through the alveolar-capillary membrane into the alveoli. The rate of diffusion depends on a low partial pressure of carbon dioxide in the alveoli. Normally, carbon dioxide makes up 0.04 percent of inspired air, and carbon dioxide from this source is also present in the alveoli. Poorly ventilated alveoli do not have this low partial pressure of carbon dioxide. Carbon dioxide diffusion does not seem to be influenced by the thickness of the alveolar-capillary membrane, probably because carbon dioxide has 10 to 20 times the diffusing capacity of oxygen. On the other hand, unless a large number of alveoli are adequately ventilated, there will be overall carbon dioxide retention.

Regulation

Normally, blood oxygen and carbon dioxide content are maintained in a relatively narrow range by adjusting the rate and depth of respiration according to body requirements for intake of oxygen and excretion of carbon dioxide. This is very similar to the way in which the rate and stroke volume of the heart are adjusted to meet the oxygen requirements of the tissues. Thus, respirations are increased by a low blood oxygen saturation and a high carbon dioxide content acting on the chemoreceptors in the carotid and aortic bodies and the respiratory center in the brain stem (B). Anoxemia is not as good a stimulus for respiration as a high carbon dioxide content (hypercapnia). Respirations may also be increased by acidosis (also acting through the carotid and aortic bodies and the respiratory center), impulses from high cortical centers, painful stimulation of the peripheral nerves, and hypotension. Respirations may be depressed by a prolonged elevation of blood carbon dioxide, prolonged anoxia, or hypertension.

Pathophysiology of Deficits and Excesses

Hypoxemia or anoxemia may result from decreased intake (laryngitis, bronchitis, emphysema), poor absorption (sarcoidosis and pulmonary edema), poor transport to the tissues (anemia, CHF) or disturbance of regulation (barbiturate intoxication, brain stem trauma, etc.).

Hyperoxemia is not associated with disease states, but may be dangerous in certain disorders (severe pulmonary emphysema, etc.).

Plasma Proteins

Intake

Proteins enter the body through the alimentary canal (A) and undergo hydrolysis to amino acids in the stomach and the small intestine. They are acted on by hydrochloric acid and pepsin in the stomach and by trypsin, chymotrypsin, and carboxypeptidase (pancreatic enzymes) as well as aminopeptidase (intestinal enzymes) in the intestinal lumen. Approximately 95 per cent of the proteins in the diet are fully digested to amino acids in this manner; only a small amount of the intermediate polypeptides are available for absorption or excretion in the feces.

Absorption

The amino acids are promptly and actively absorbed by the small intestine (B); virtually none pass into the feces normally.

Production

Following their absorption, the amino acids are transported by the blood to the liver, the reticuloendothelial system, and all the other body cells in which formation of proteins takes place. Of the proteins circulating in the blood, albumin, the alpha and beta globulins, prothrombin, and fibrinogen are all formed in the liver. The gamma globulins are not exclusively of hepatic origin but are synthesized in all the reticuloendothelial tissues of the body. A 70-Kg. man produces and degrades about 15 to 20 gm. of plasma protein a day in maintaining a dynamic equilibrium.

The average adult requires 0.5 gm. of protein per kilogram per day, including certain essential amino acids.

Transport and Functions

Once synthesized, the plasma proteins are released into the blood stream to assume their various metabolic roles. Normally, there is 6 to 8 gm. of plasma protein per 100 ml. of blood (C). Electrophoretic analysis has shown that 100 ml. of blood contains 3.5 to 5.1 gm. of albumin, 0.7 to 1.5 gm. of alpha globulin, 0.7 to 1.3 gm. of beta globulin, and 0.7 to 1.5 gm. of gamma globulin.

These proteins have many useful functions in the body. They serve as a source of protein nutrition for the tissues during protein deprivation. They serve as buffers for acid-base balance. One of their most important roles is maintaining the normal distribution of water in the organism. This function is performed primarily by the albumin fraction, which is responsible for about 80 percent of the oncotic pressure of human plasma. As plasma protein decreases, plasma water decreases and vice versa. At the same time extracellular fluid (edema) increases or decreases.

Equally important is their role in transporting other constituents of the blood. Thus plasma lipids, vitamins, steroid and thyroid hormones, metals (iron, copper, etc.), and certain enzymes are carried by the blood proteins.

The gamma globulins contain the all-important antibodies (to typhoid, mumps, poliomyelitis, etc.). Fibrinogen, prothrombin, and a number of other plasma proteins participate in coagulation.

Storage

Unlike fat, stored protein cannot be assigned to any particular cell. However, all body cells, particularly those of the liver, kidney, and intestines, possess labile proteins that can be metabolized during starvation to meet the caloric requirements of the organism[8] (D).

Destruction

The plasma proteins, as indicated above, may be broken down to amino acids by the liver and utilized by the body either as energy or in the formation of substances essential to the body such as enzymes, hormones (insulin, etc.), and purines or pyrimidines for the production of new cells. Amino acids are utilized for energy by deamination to such substances as pyruvic acid (formed from alanine), alpha-ketoglutaric acid (formed from glutamic acid), and aspartic acid and introduced into the Krebs cycle. The end products of protein catabolism are urea, carbon dioxide, water, uric acid, phosphates, and creatinine (E).

Excretion

Only minimal amounts of protein and amino acids are excreted normally. The quantities that are filtered

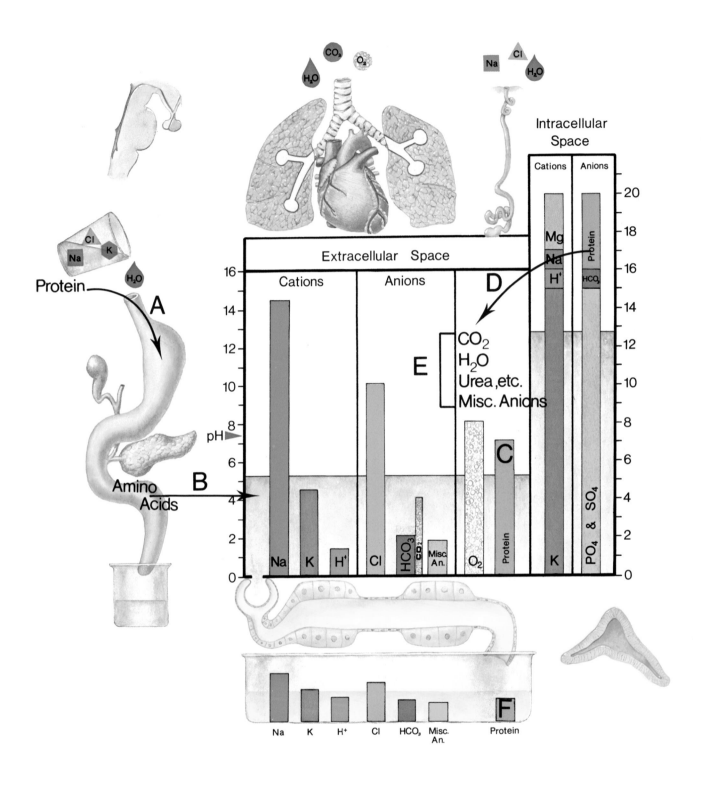

through the glomeruli are almost completely reabsorbed. However, both amino acids and protein appear in the urine in a variety of pathologic conditions (F). The degradation products of protein (urea, carbon dioxide, water, etc.) are, of course, excreted in the urine and through the lungs. These are discussed elsewhere.

Regulation

The plasma proteins, and in fact all the body proteins, are constantly being broken down to amino acids and then resynthesized. All the factors influencing this equilibrium are not known, but among them are the quantity and the quality of amino acids in the diet, the metabolic rate, and certain hormones, the most important of which are growth hormone, corticosteroids, androgens, thyroid hormone, and insulin. Growth hormone, androgens, and insulin increase protein synthesis, whereas glucocorticoids and large amounts of thyroid increase protein catabolism. There is some evidence that growth hormone and insulin act synergistically in promoting protein synthesis. Physiologic amounts of both corticosteroids and thyroid hormone exert an anabolic effect on protein metabolism.

Pathophysiology of Deficits and Excesses

Hypoproteinemia may result from decreased intake (malnutrition), decreased absorption (malabsorption syndrome), decreased production (cirrhosis of the liver), abnormal excretion (nephrotic syndrome) and hemodilution (congestive heart failure).

Hyperproteinemia results from increased production (as in multiple myeloma) and hemoconcentration (dehydration).

Section Two

Effects of Individual
Fluid and Electrolyte Alterations

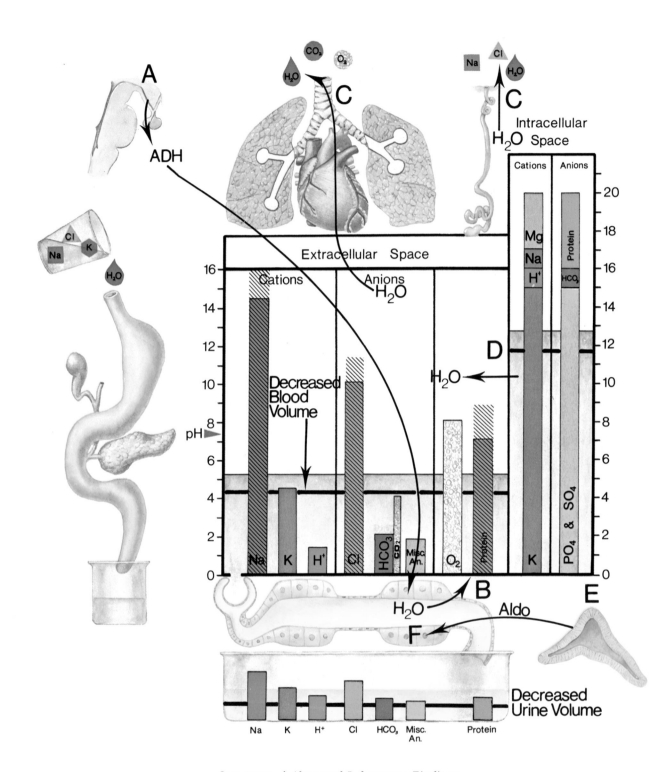

Summary of Abnormal Laboratory Findings

Serum Na—increased

Serum K—normal or
    decreased

Serum Cl—increased

Serum HCO_3^-—normal
    or increased

Serum protein—
    increased

Blood volume—
    decreased*

Urine volume—
    decreased

Water Deficiency

Pathophysiology

When there is restriction of water intake, the concentrations of serum *sodium* and *chloride rise* and the consequent hyperosmolality stimulates the supraoptic nucleus (A) to release ADH. This increases the permeability of the distal and collecting tubules to water and much of it is reabsorbed (B). However, there is a limit to the kidney's ability to conserve water as it continues to put out 500 to 600 ml. of urine a day. Furthermore, insensible water loss (600-800 ml. a day) continues to be lost via the lungs and skin (C). Sweat production (sensible water loss) becomes negligible. The hypertonic plasma and extracellular fluid compensate further by drawing water from the cells (D). Nevertheless *blood volume* remains *low*. This stimulates the juxtaglomerular cells to secrete renin, activating angiotensin and the release of aldosterone from the adrenal cortex (E). This acts on the distal tubule (F) to conserve sodium. However, potassium and hydrogen ion are lost in the process. Thus a *hypokalemic* metabolic alkalosis may result. Some sodium and chloride continue to be lost in the urine.

Clinical Picture

There is loss of eyeball tension and skin turgor and the mucous membranes and tongue are dry. The temperature and pulse may be elevated, but the blood pressure may drop. In late stages delirium and coma may result.

Diagnosis

The high serum sodium and chloride with a normal or low potassium are almost diagnostic. Hematocrit and plasma protein are elevated, but blood volume is low. Spinal fluid pressure is invariably low. Both plasma and urine osmolality are increased.

Etiology

Water deficit is the major alteration in dehydration, diabetes insipidus, hyperosmolar nonketotic diabetic coma, nephrogenic diabetes insipidus and certain cases of chronic pyelonephritis. Comparison of the plasma and urine osmolality help differentiate pure dehydration from renal disease and diabetes insipidus. In dehydration the ratio of urine to plasma osmolality will be greater than 1:1.

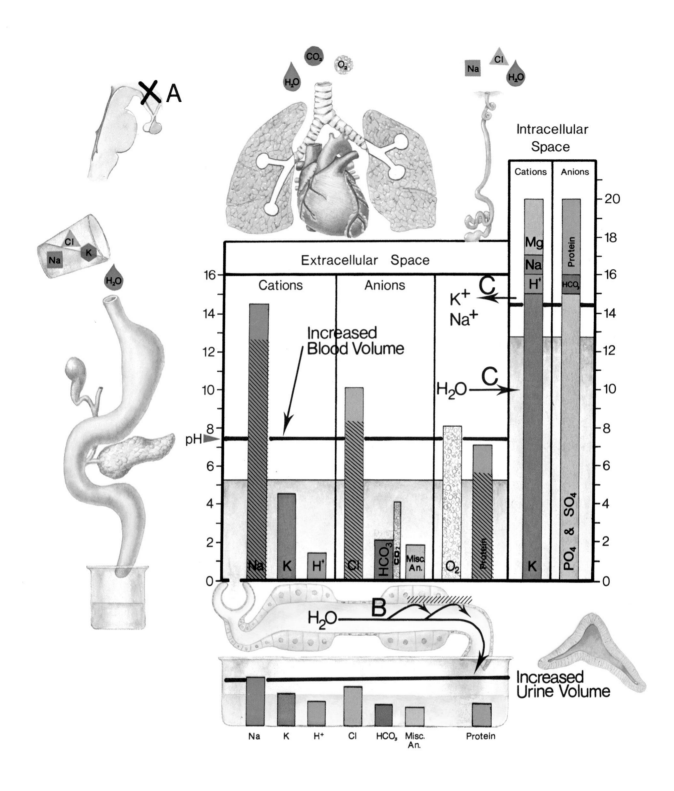

Summary of Abnormal Laboratory Findings

Serum Na—decreased

Serum Cl—decreased

Serum protein—
 decreased

Blood volume—
 increased*

Urine volume—
 increased

Water Excess

Pathophysiology

If large amounts of 5 percent dextrose and water are administered to normal subjects *blood volume* will *increase** and serum *sodium* and *chloride* concentrations will *drop*. The resulting hypotonicity of the serum inhibits the secretion of ADH by the supraoptic nucleus (A). Thus reabsorption of water from the distal and collecting tubules is diminished (B) and *urine volume increases* while blood volume is returned to normal. Unless the fluid is administered very rapidly, very little increase in sodium and chloride excretion will occur so that the urine osmolality will be low. Water enters the cells and cellular electrolytes (potassium etc.) may move extracellularly (C) to compensate for the serum hypotonicity (decreased osmolality). *Cellular volume* increases, but cellular electrolyte concentrations decrease.

Clinical Picture

There may be abdominal or skeletal muscular twitching or cramping, stupor and convulsions. Pulmonary and peripheral edema may develop in severe cases. Fingerprinting of the skin indicates intracellular volume excess.

Diagnosis

Low serum sodium and chloride, increased blood and urine volume with a decreased serum and urine osmolality are very helpful signs. Serum protein and hematocrit will also be lower than normal.

Etiology

Water excess is found most often in acute congestive heart failure, acute renal failure, pathologic diaphoresis and inappropriate ADH secretion.

---

*Hereafter the blood volume changes will be indicated by an asterisk in the illustrations.

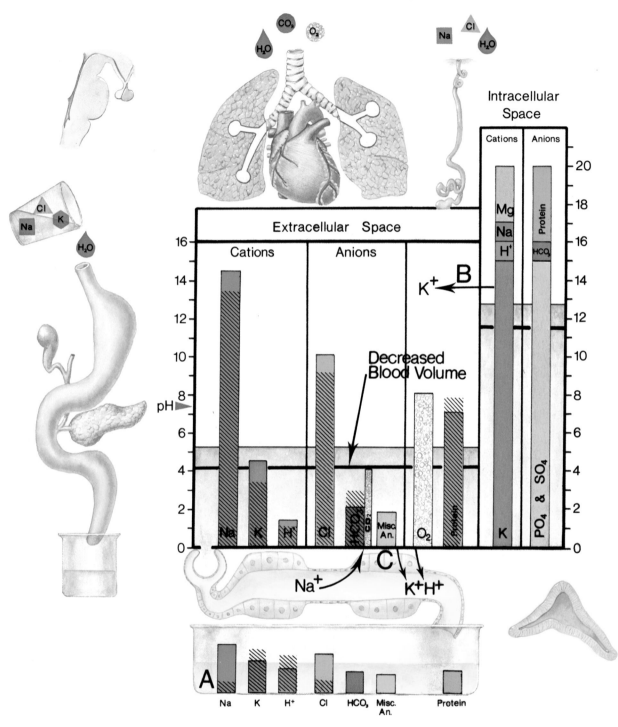

Summary of Abnormal Laboratory Findings

Serum Na—decreased
Serum K—normal or
    decreased
Serum H⁺—decreased
    or normal
Serum Cl—decreased
Serum HCO₃⁻—normal
    or increased

Serum protein—
    increased
Blood volume—
    decreased*
Urine volume—
    increased, normal
    or decreased

Sodium Chloride Deficiency

Pathophysiology

Patients placed on a low salt diet will not develop a reduced serum sodium and chloride immediately. The kidney has such a remarkable ability to conserve sodium that it can drop the concentration of sodium and chloride in the urine (A) to almost zero (10 mEq./L.). After four or five days the *serum sodium and chloride will drop* and since sodium and chloride deficits are accompanied by water deficits in the normal individual the *blood volume will also drop*. This is because hyponatremia (and consequent hypotonicity) inhibits the release of ADH. To delay this development fluid and electrolytes, particularly potassium, will move out of the cell (B) to maintain plasma volume. The reduced plasma volume stimulates the release of aldosterone through the renin-angiotensin system (discussed on page 9). This enhances the reabsorption of sodium in exchange for potassium and hydrogen ion (C). Thus *serum potassium and hydrogen ion drops* and a metabolic alkalosis may ensue. If sodium restriction is allowed to continue, the hyponatremia will be compensated for by a shift of water back into the cells. At this point urine output will have made a significant drop.

Clinical Picture

Clinical symptoms and signs may not develop until serum sodium drops below 115 mEq./L. At that point water moves into the cells, the sensorium becomes clouded and seizures or coma may develop.

Diagnosis

To differentiate a pure sodium or salt depletion from dilutional hyponatremia, blood volume, hematocrit, and serum protein should be measured. Hematocrit and serum protein will be *increased* in pure sodium or salt deficit, but decreased in dilutional hyponatremia. The blood volume will show the reverse.

Etiology

Decreased salt intake is unusual, but decreased absorption may occur in diarrhea, malabsorption syndrome and severe vomiting. Increased excretion (resulting in the above picture) may occur in diabetic acidosis, chronic renal disease, excessive sweating (without water replacement) and adrenal insufficiency.

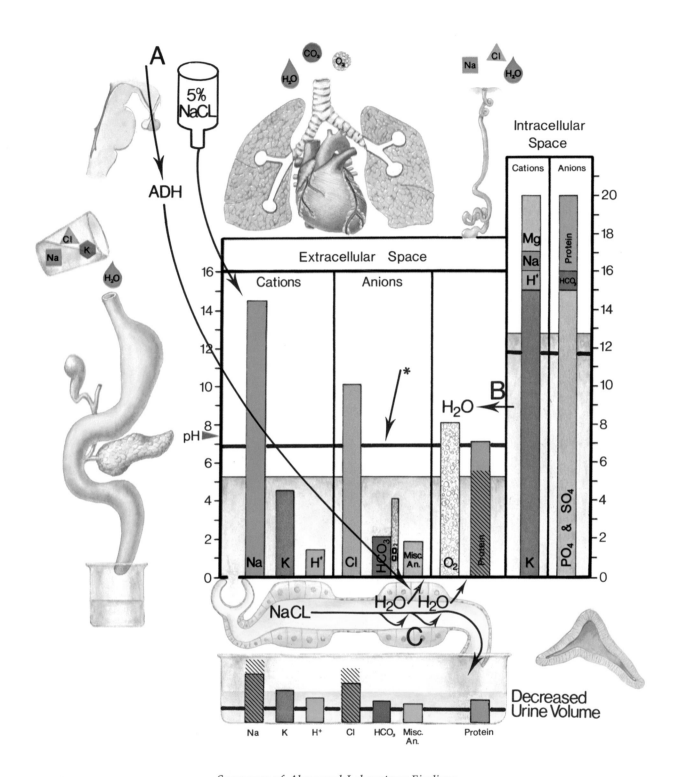

Summary of Abnormal Laboratory Findings

Serum Na—normal or
    increased

Serum Cl—normal or
    increased

Serum protein—
    decreased

Blood volume—
    increased*

Urine volume—
    decreased or
    normal

Sodium Chloride Excess

Pathophysiology

What will happen if a hypertonic solution of sodium chloride is given orally or intravenously to the normal subject? Serum sodium and chloride will increase temporarily. The increased tonicity will stimulate the supraoptic nucleus (A) to secrete ADH and enhance the reabsorption of water from the distal and collecting tubules reestablishing normal plasma tonicity but *increasing volume*. Water will also move out of the cells (B) enhancing the *increase in blood volume*. The increased blood volume will subsequently inhibit aldosterone secretion by way of the renin-angiotensin system (described on page 9) and distal renal tubular reabsorption of sodium in exchange for hydrogen and potassium will decrease (C). Proximal tubular reabsorption of sodium is also reduced by an as yet undefined mechanism.[9] For this and other reasons the excess *sodium and chloride are excreted in the urine* and gradually the blood volume returns to normal.

Clinical Picture

Symptoms are rather mild but edema and congestive heart failure may develop, particularly in the elderly.

Diagnosis

Increased blood volume will be the most helpful diagnostic study since the rises in serum sodium and chloride will be transitory.

Etiology

Excessive intake of salt may occur during intravenous therapy (isotonic saline is acutally hypertonic, containing 154 mEq. Na/L.) and during hyperalimentation either orally or intravenously. Excessive retention of salt may occur in a variety of disorders (see both Hypernatremia and Hyponatremia in Table 3).

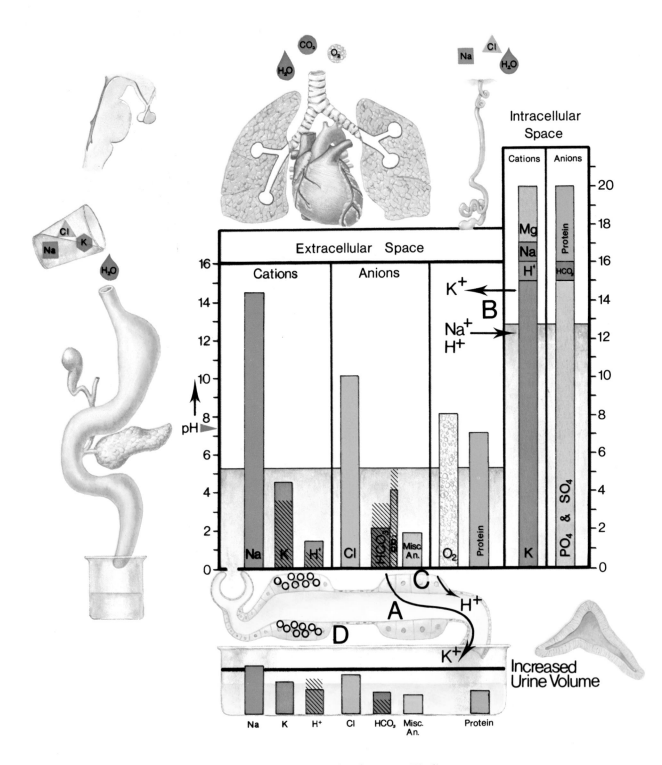

Intracellular Space

Extracellular Space

Summary of Abnormal Laboratory Findings

Serum K—decreased
Serum H^+—decreased
Serum HCO_3^-—increased
Blood PCO_2—increased or normal

Blood pH—increased
Urine H^+—increased
Urine HCO_3^-—decreased
Urine volume—increased

Potassium Deficiency

Pathophysiology

Potassium restriction soon leads to a *drop in serum potassium* because the kidneys continue to excrete 40 to 50 mEq. a day for some time (A). Compensatory mechanisms take place, but generally fail to bring the serum potassium level back to normal. Potassium moves out of the cell in exchange for sodium and hydrogen ion (B). The *serum hydrogen ion* drops and a metabolic alkalosis results. This is further aggravated by the preferential secretion of hydrogen ion (which is more available than potassium) by the distal tubule in exchange for sodium (C). Thus, the urine is generally slightly acid in these subjects. In long-standing potassium depletion there is vacuolization of the proximal convoluted tubules (D) and dilatation of the collecting tubules.[10] These patients lose their ability to concentrate the urine because of inability to respond to ADH.[3]

Clinical Picture

There may be clouding of the sensorium, muscular weakness, hyporeflexia and even frank flaccid paralysis of the extremities. Intestinal mobility is decreased and a paralytic ileus may be observed. Bradycardia, heart block and other arrhythmias may occur. The EKG may show ST depression, inversion of the T-waves and falsely prolonged Q-T interval because of prominent U-waves. The P-R interval may also be prolonged.

Diagnosis

The serum potassium and EKG changes are essential for the diagnosis.

Etiology

See Table 3.

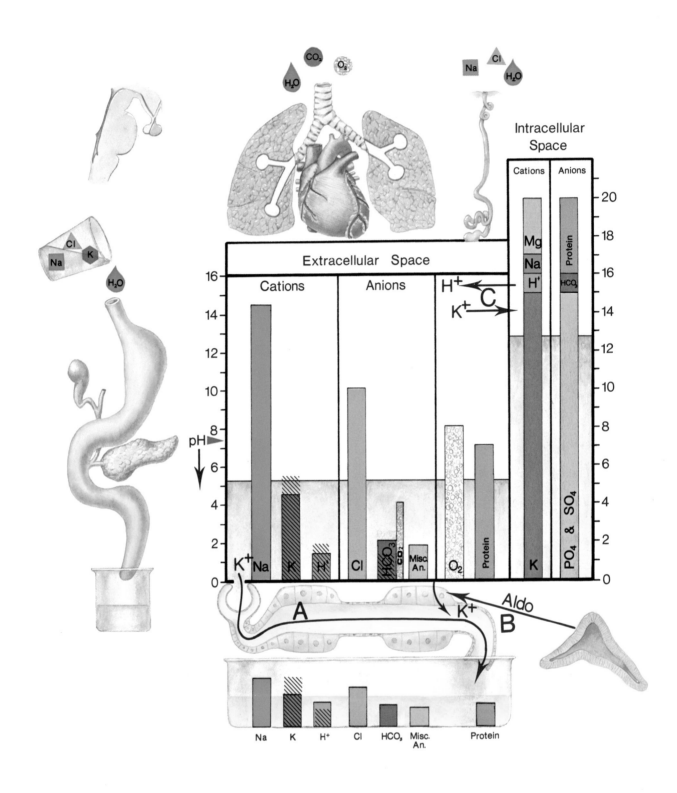

Summary of Abnormal Laboratory Findings

Serum K—increased   Blood pH—decreased
Serum H⁺—increased   Urine K—increased
Serum HCO₃⁻—   Urine H⁺—decreased
   decreased

Potassium Excess

Pathophysiology

Rapid administration of potassium intravenously will cause the serum potassium to rise. The excess potassium is soon excreted by the kidneys (A) both because of a solute diuresis and because the hyperkalemia stimulates the adrenal cortex to release aldosterone.[11] This acts on the distal tubule (B) to enhance the secretion of potassium in exchange for sodium. Less *hydrogen ion* will be secreted and its blood level *rises* leading to a metabolic acidosis. In addition potassium moves into the cell and hydrogen ion moves out (C) adding to the acidosis.

Clinical Picture

Hyperkalemia rarely induces changes in the sensorium such as anxiety, agitation and later stupor.

Severe weakness, hyporeflexia and even paralysis of the extremities may result. The most serious effect is on the heart. In the early stages there are peaked T-waves. Subsequently there is widening of the QRS and P-R interval. Then heart block may occur or various arrhythmias including ventricular fibrillation. There may be sudden cardiac arrest in diastole.

Diagnosis

This is best determined by the serum potassium and EKG changes.

Etiology

Most cases of hyperkalemia are due to renal failure, spironolactone diuretics or Addison's disease. Others are listed in Table 3.

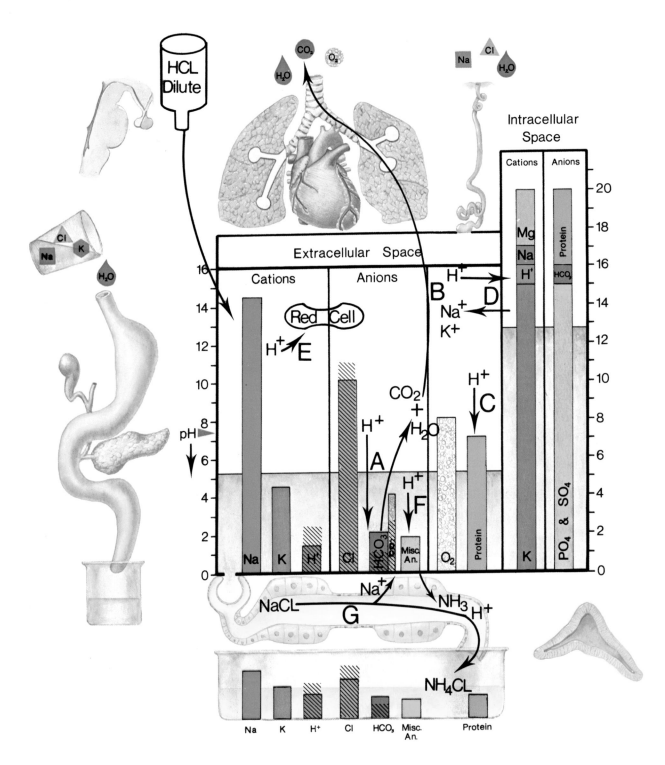

Summary of Abnormal Laboratory Findings

Serum K—increased or normal

Serum H⁺—increased

Serum Cl—increased

Serum HCO₃⁻—decreased

Blood Pco₂—decreased

Blood pH—decreased

Urine K—increased or normal

Urine H⁺—increased

Urine Cl—increased

Urine HCO₃⁻—decreased

Urine volume—increased

Acid Excess

Pathophysiology

Let's suppose that a dilute solution of HCl were infused into the blood. What would happen? The hydrogen would be neutralized in several ways because the body is well equipped to handle acidosis. It may combine with HCO_3^- (A) to produce the weaker acid H_2CO_3 which would split into H_2O and CO_2 in the lungs and allow for the CO_2 to escape reducing the acidity of the blood in this fashion (B). Respirations may be increased to blow off the excess CO_2. It may combine with the plasma protein (C), to form a weaker acid and release Na^+ or K^+ which could be rebound later. It may enter the cell (D) in exchange for Na^+ and K^+ and bind with cellular protein, phosphates or sulfates to form weaker acids. It may enter the red cell (E) and be buffered by the hemoglobin. It may also combine with the phosphate buffer system (F) (miscellaneous anions) transforming Na_2HPO_4 to NaH_2PO_4.

The *chloride increases* the concentration of plasma chloride momentarily, but this is later excreted in the glomerular filtrate as NaCl (G). Then the tubular cells, by forming NH_3 from glutamine and H_2CO_3 from H_2O and CO_2 under the influence of carbonic anhydrase make a characteristic swap in regenerating bicarbonate. Na^+ is reabsorbed with the HCO_3^- from the tubular cell (H) and H^+ is joined to NH_3 and Cl^- to be excreted as NH_4Cl. Once enough sodium bicarbonate is regenerated by the kidneys in this fashion the plasma electrolytes are returned to normal and they can begin accepting hydrogen ion back from plasma protein, phosphates, the intracellular fluids and the red cells.

Clinical Picture

Hyperventilation, clouded sensorium and coma may occur. Occasionally there may be signs of dehydration and abdominal pain.

Diagnosis

Serum electrolytes and arterial blood gases will establish the diagnosis.

Etiology

Ammonium chloride administration commonly produces this picture, but ingestion of any acid may cause it also.

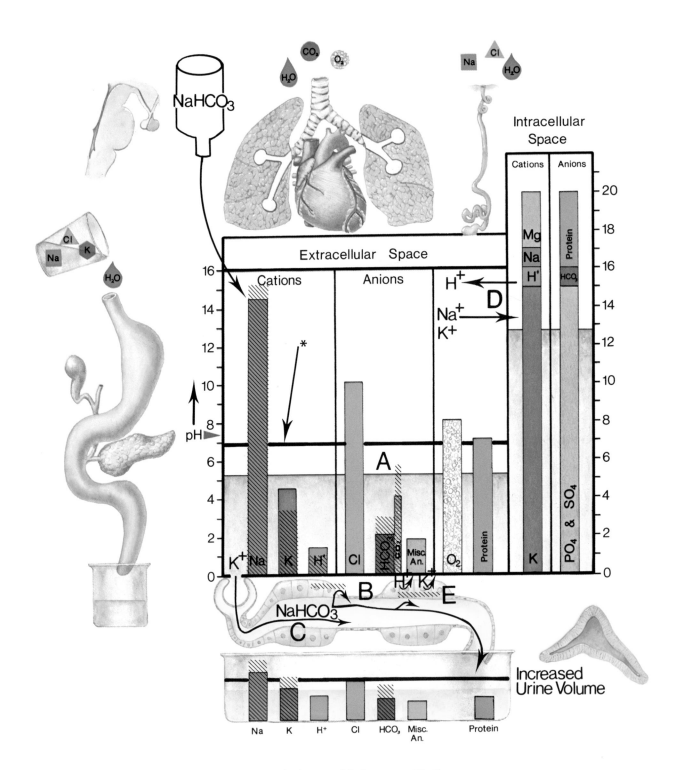

Summary of Abnormal Laboratory Findings

Serum Na—increased

Serum K—decreased

Serum H⁺—decreased

Serum HCO₃⁻—increased

Blood Pco₂—increased

Blood pH—increased

Blood volume—
  increased*

Urine Na—increased

Urine K—increased

Urine volume—
  increased

Sodium Bicarbonate Excess

Pathophysiology

When sodium bicarbonate is administered orally or by infusion, the blood levels of each ion *rise* and a metabolic alkalosis develops. Then compensatory mechanisms come into play. Respirations are reduced with consequent *rise in* P_{CO_2} (A) and carbonic acid. The kidney excretes larger amounts of sodium bicarbonate because proximal tubular reabsorption is inhibited (B). There is *increased excretion of potassium* in the *urine* (C) to help eliminate the bicarbonate. However, the potassium deficit, if too great, aggravates the alkalosis because hydrogen ions are secreted instead of potassium to reabsorb sodium from the distal tubular lumen. Sodium and potassium move into the cell (D) in exchange for hydrogen ion. The infusion of sodium bicarbonate will *increase blood volume,* suppressing the release of renin from the juxtaglomerular apparatus and consequently cause a reduction in aldosterone secretion. This will reduce the secretion of both potassium and hydrogen ion in exchange for sodium by the distal tubule (E) and further compensate for the metabolic alkalosis.

Clinical Picture

In addition to the symptoms and signs of hypokalemia, there will be depressed respirations and ultimately stupor and coma. There may be tetany and convulsions as a result of the decrease in ionized calcium.

Diagnosis

The serum electrolyte changes together with a pH (elevated) will be diagnostic.

Etiology

This picture can be seen when excessive sodium bicarbonate is given in treating diabetic acidosis and cardiac arrest. It is also seen when there is too vigorous treatment of respiratory acidosis.

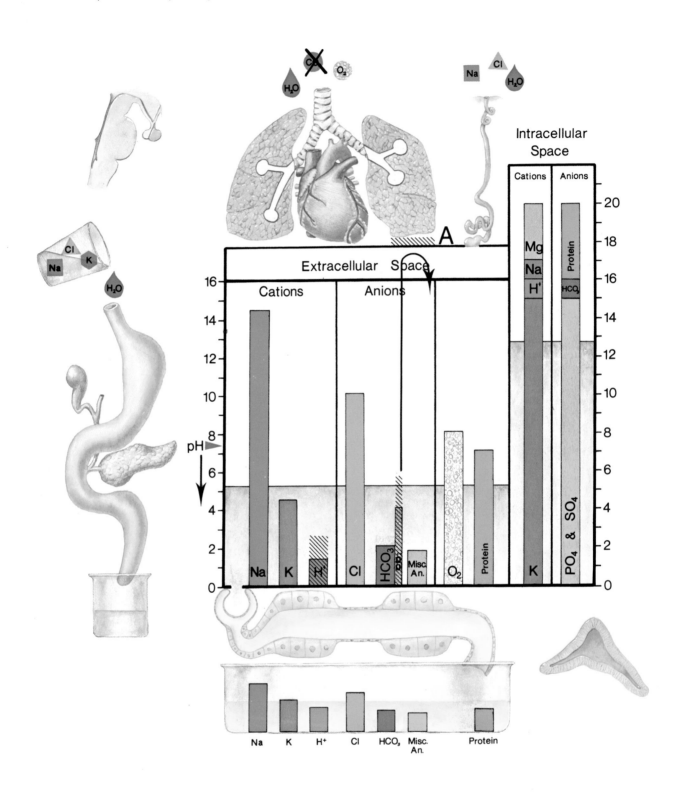

Summary of Abnormal Laboratory Findings
Blood P_{CO_2}—increased
Serum H^+—increased
Blood pH—decreased

Uncompensated Respiratory Acidosis

Alveolar hypoventilation as occurs in pulmonary emphysema, acute bronchial asthma and other forms of obstructive lung disease at first results in decreased carbon dioxide excretion via the lungs (A). Thus the blood P_{CO_2} and *carbonic acid increase. Hydrogen ion increases* and *pH drops.* This is uncompensated respiratory acidosis.

Clinical Picture

Hyperventilation, clouded sensorium, rapid pulse and occasional cyanosis and coma are the usual findings.

Diagnosis

This is established by serum electrolytes, arterial blood gases and pulmonary function tests.

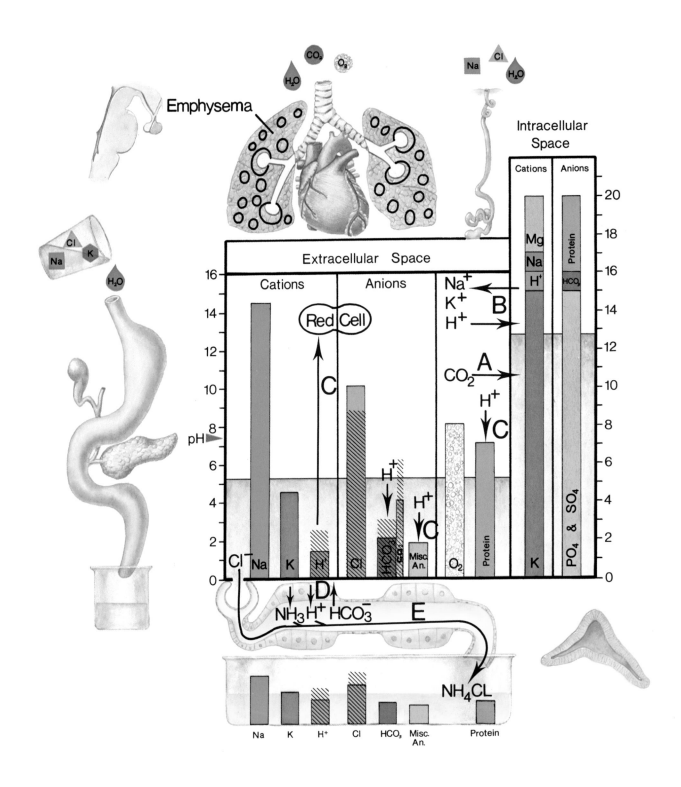

Summary of Abnormal Laboratory Findings
Blood P$_{CO_2}$—increased
Serum H$^+$—increased
  or normal
Serum HCO$_3^-$—
  increased

Serum Cl—decreased
Blood pH—normal or
  only slightly
  decreased

Compensated Respiratory Acidosis

In chronic alveolar hypoventilation from pulmonary emphysema and bronchial asthma the blood P_{CO_2} and carbonic acid increase, but compensatory mechanisms are brought into play to *restore the pH to normal.* Respirations increase to assist the escape of carbon dioxide. Some of the carbon dioxide passes into the cell (A) and is buffered by the cellular protein, phosphates, etc. Hydrogen ions formed from the carbonic acid ($H_2O + CO_2 \rightarrow H^+ + HCO_3^-$) move into the cell in exchange for sodium and potassium (B). Hydrogen ion is buffered by the red cells and the plasma and extracellular bicarbonate, phosphates and protein (C). There is increased reabsorption of bicarbonate by the kidneys (D) in exchange for the secretion of hydrogen ion in the tubules. Thus *serum bicarbonate increases.* The hydrogen ion secreted into the renal tubules combines with ammonium and chloride and is excreted into the urine (E). Since large amounts of *chloride* may be needed to excrete the hydrogen ion, its *serum level drops.*

Clinical Picture

Hyperventilation, tachycardia, clouded sensorium, occasional coma, cyanosis, clubbing and polycythemia are the usual features. The lungs show hyperresonance, diminished alveolar breath sounds, and sibilant and sonorous rales in emphysema.

Diagnosis

This is established by serum electrolytes, arterial blood gases and pulmonary function studies.

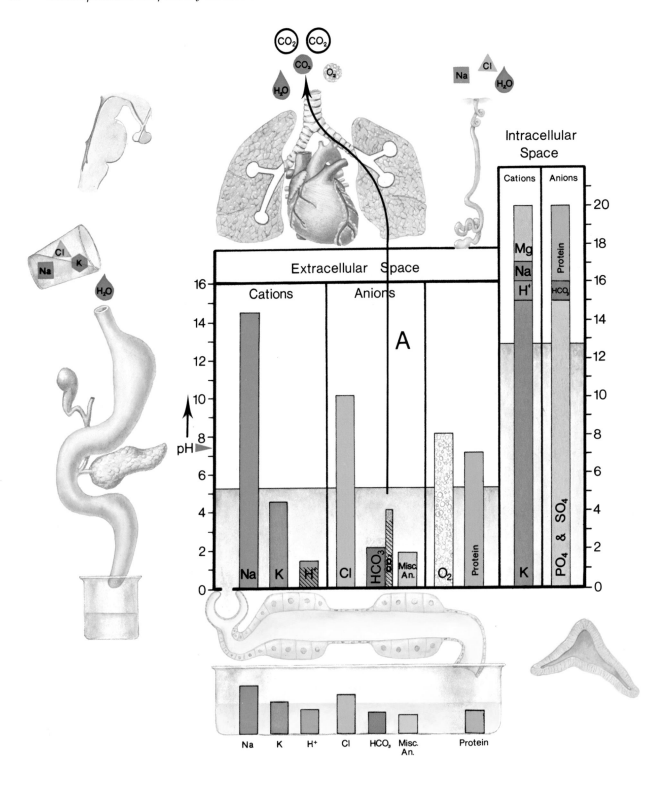

Summary of Abnormal Laboratory Findings
Blood P_{CO_2}—decreased
Serum H^+—decreased
Blood pH—increased

Uncompensated Respiratory Alkalosis

Hyperventilation as occurs in salicylate intoxication, anxiety, pulmonary embolism, shock and many central nervous system diseases increases the excretion of carbon dioxide through the lungs (A). Thus *blood* P_{CO_2}, *hydrogen ion,* and *carbonic acid drop* while *pH rises.*

Clinical Picture

Hyperventilation, clouded sensorium and occasional coma, tachycardia and a drop in blood pressure may occur. Tetany may result from the decrease in ionized calcium.

Diagnosis

Serum electrolytes and arterial blood gases establish the diagnosis in most cases.

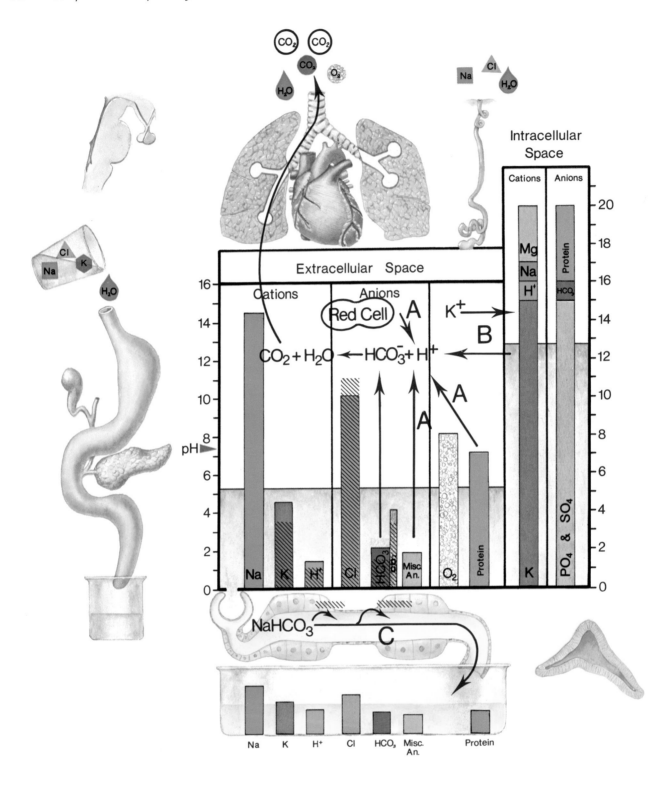

Summary of Abnormal Laboratory Findings

Blood P_{CO_2}—decreased
Serum H^+—decreased
   or normal
Serum
   HCO_3^-—decreased

Serum K—decreased
Serum Cl—increased
Blood pH—normal or
   only slightly
   increased

Compensated Respiratory Alkalosis

If the hyperventilation in salicylate intoxication (page 129) and other disorders continues, the *blood* P_{CO_2} and *hydrogen ion decrease,* but compensatory mechanisms are brought into play to restore the pH to normal. Bicarbonate is converted to carbonic acid by receiving hydrogen ion from the red cells (hemoglobin), plasma protein and extracellular phosphate buffers (A) and the intracellular buffers (mainly protein). Therefore *serum bicarbonate drops. Potassium* moves into the cell in exchange for hydrogen ion (B) and its *plasma level falls.* The kidney excretes more bicarbonate (C) because there is less potassium and hydrogen ion to secrete in exchange for sodium bicarbonate. More chloride is reabsorbed because less is needed for hydrogen ion excretion. Thus *serum chloride* may be *elevated.*

Clinical Picture

As in uncompensated respiratory alkalosis.

Diagnosis

This is established by serum electrolytes and arterial blood gases.

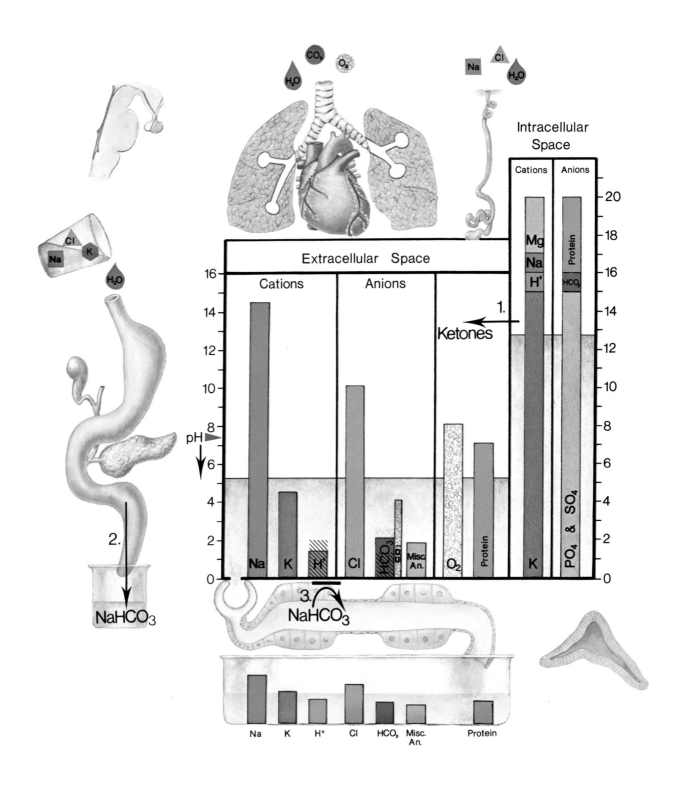

Summary of Abnormal Laboratory Findings
Serum H^+—increased
Serum HCO_3^-—
    decreased
Blood pH—decreased

Uncompensated Metabolic Acidosis

Pathophysiology

This condition results under three circumstances:
1. When an acid other than carbonic acid pours into or accumulates in the system (acetoacetic acid of diabetic ketosis, etc.).
2. When there is excessive loss of bicarbonate (as in diarrhea).
3. When the kidney's ability to form or reabsorb bicarbonate is impaired (as in renal tubular acidosis). In all cases the serum *hydrogen ion increases* and the *serum bicarbonate* and *blood pH drops*.

Clinical Picture

There is usually hyperventilation, clouding of the sensorium progressing to coma, often signs of dehydration and occasional abdominal pain. Other signs are compatible with the cause of the metabolic acidosis.

Diagnosis

The *low serum bicarbonate* and *blood pH* are diagnostic. A low P_{CO_2} will not be present unless compensatory mechanisms have begun (see page 57).

Etiology

See Table 3 under "Decreased Bicarbonate."

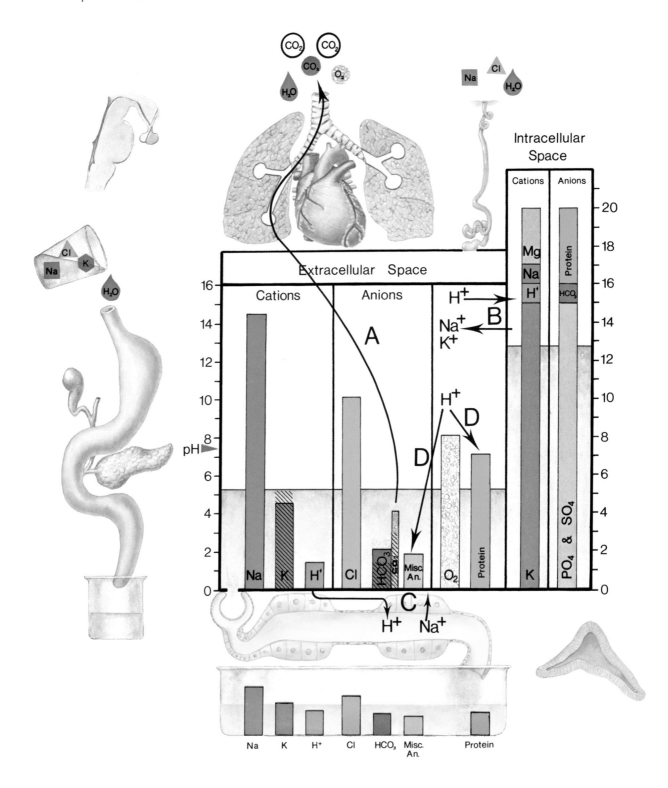

Summary of Abnormal Laboratory Findings

Serum H^+—increased or normal

Serum HCO_3^-— decreased

Blood pH—low normal or slight decrease

Blood P_{CO_2}—decreased

Serum potassium— increased or normal

Compensated Metabolic Acidosis

Pathophysiology

This condition occurs under the same circumstances as the uncompensated form. The *serum hydrogen ion increases* while the serum bicarbonate decreases, but certain compensatory mechanisms are brought into play to keep the *blood pH normal* or near normal. There is hyperventilation with increased excretion of carbon dioxide via the lungs (A) and *blood P_{CO_2} drops*. Hydrogen ion enters the cell in exchange for Na and K ions (B). This will often cause a rise in serum potassium. More hydrogen ion is secreted by the distal tubule (C) in exchange for sodium (which is reabsorbed as bicarbonate rather than chloride). This last compensatory mechanism will not occur in renal tubular acidosis and chronic renal disease. The hydrogen ion is buffered by plasma protein, phosphate buffers (in miscellaneous anions) (D) and red cells. Skeletal sodium seems also to be available for exchange with hydrogen ions.[12]

Clinical Picture

As in uncompensated metabolic acidosis.

Diagnosis

The serum electrolytes will show the low bicarbonate and often an elevation of potassium. If the condition is due to diabetic ketoacidosis or lactic acidosis, these will be elevated and there will be a characteristic anion gap. If the condition is due to diarrhea or renal tubular acidosis, the serum chloride may be elevated. Blood gases will show a low P_{CO_2} and low or low normal pH.

Etiology

See Table 3 under "Decreased Bicarbonate."

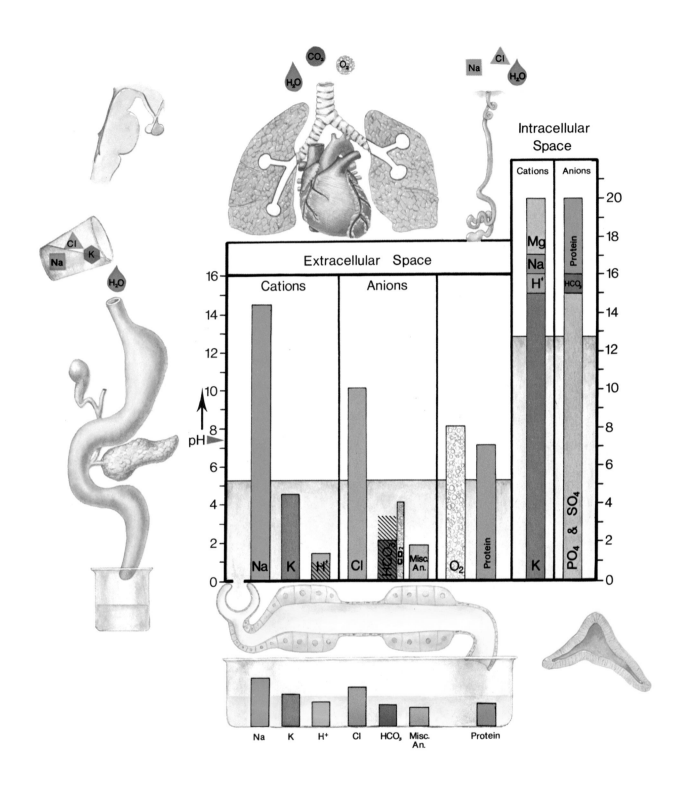

Summary of Abnormal Laboratory Findings
Serum H+—decreased
Serum HCO₃⁻—
    increased
Blood pH—increased

Uncompensated Metabolic Alkalosis

Pathophysiology

This condition results from loss of fixed acid (as in vomiting or nasogastric suction), ingestion or administration of alkali (sodium bicarbonate, etc.), increased production of sodium bicarbonate by the kidney under the influence of hormones (aldosterone, etc.), or diuretics (mercurials), and potassium depletion forcing the kidney to secrete more hydrogen ion in exchange for sodium bicarbonate. There is an *increase* of *serum bicarbonate* without an accompanying increase in carbon dioxide and carbonic acid, an *increase* in *blood pH* and a *decrease* in *hydrogen ion.*

Clinical Picture

Tetany with associated muscular twitching and cramping and convulsions are the main clinical features. The tetany is due to a decrease in ionized calcium. Since there is usually an associated hypokalemia, signs of this (page 39) may also be present.

Diagnosis

Serum electrolytes will show an *increased bicarbonate* and arterial blood gas analysis will show an *increased pH.*

Etiology

In addition to those conditions listed above, metabolic alkalosis may occur in all the conditions listed in Table 3 under "Increased Bicarbonate," except pulmonary emphysema and other forms of respiratory acidosis.

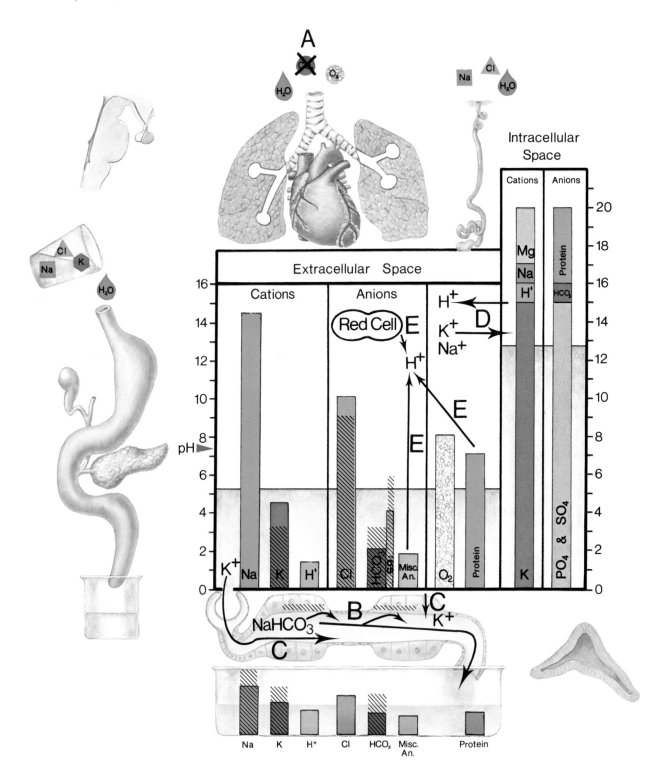

Summary of Abnormal Laboratory Findings

Serum H⁺—decreased

Serum K—decreased

Serum HCO₃⁻—
increased

Serum Cl—usually
decreased

Blood pH—normal or
slightly increased

Blood Pco₂—increased

Compensated Metabolic Alkalosis

Pathophysiology

As in uncompensated metabolic alkalosis the *serum bicarbonate increases* whereas the *serum hydrogen ion decreases*, but certain compensatory mechanisms are brought into play to maintain the *blood pH at normal* or near normal levels. There is hypoventilation with a decrease in carbon dioxide excretion (A) and a consequent *rise in P_{CO_2}* and carbonic acid. However the P_{CO_2} rarely rises above 60 mm. Hg (helping to distinguish this from respiratory acidosis[2]). The kidney excretes larger amounts of sodium bicarbonate (B) because proximal and distal tubular reabsorption is inhibited by the decrease in hydrogen ion available for this exchange. There is increased excretion of potassium in the urine (C) to help eliminate bicarbonate. This plus the movement of potassium into the cell (D) in exchange for hydrogen ion leads to a *low serum potassium*. Sodium also moves into the cell in exchange for hydrogen ion (D). Potassium is also secreted preferentially by the distal tubule (because hydrogen ion is less available) in exchange for sodium which is usually reabsorbed as sodium chloride to maintain plasma volume. In cases in which the metabolic acidosis is due to a loss of chloride (vomiting and nasogastric suction) the *serum chloride will be reduced* considerably. Finally, hydrogen ion is released from the protein, red cell and phosphate buffers of the blood to compensate further (E).

Clinical Picture

Tetany will be the main clinical feature as described in uncompensated metabolic alkalosis.

Diagnosis

The serum electrolytes will show the *increased bicarbonate* and decreased potassium and chloride. Arterial blood gas analysis will show the increased P_{CO_2} and this with the higher pH differentiates this condition from compensated respiratory acidosis.

Etiology

Compensated metabolic alkalosis may occur in all those conditions listed in Table 3 except pulmonary emphysema and other forms of respiratory acidosis.

Section Three

The Diagnosis of Fluid and Electrolyte Disorders

The usual approach to any type of diagnosis is taking a history, doing a physical examination and ordering laboratory work to support or rule out the diagnostic possibilities suggested by the history and the physical. This is fine when one has an alert, cooperative patient and there is plenty of time. The reader is well aware that in electrolyte disorders this frequently is not the case. The patient may be comatose and a real medical emergency may exist that demands immediate treatment.

Consequently another approach is presented here. Given the laboratory serum electrolyte report, what are the diagnostic possibilities? First the report should be examined for accuracy. This can be determined by calculating the anion gap (page 162). If this is normal, the laboratory report is less in doubt. If the anion gap is high, there should be clinical and other electrolyte data to support a metabolic acidosis or renal failure; if not, the electrolyte determination should be repeated. If the report is valid, it should fit with the clinical picture. Table 1 shows the signs and symptoms to be expected with various alterations.

Sometimes this is all that is needed, especially when there is a good history.

Frequently the data in electrolytes do not fit the clinical picture. Table 2 may help in these cases. This table gives the typical electrolyte changes in common clinical disorders. If the combination of changes does not fit any of these disorders, Table 4 should be consulted. This will give the differential diagnosis of all the possible combinations. It is arranged in three sections: hypernatremia, normonatremia and hyponatremia. Once a list of possibilities is obtained from this table, the clinical picture can be reexamined, a definitive diagnosis may then be possible and additional laboratory work (mentioned in Table 4) ordered to confirm it. Often a blood gas determination (especially for the pH) will suggest the diagnosis. Table 5 will assist the clinician in interpreting this. When only single alterations are found in the electrolyte report, Table 3 will provide a list of possibilities. Section Six provides the reader with several exercises in the use of these tables. It is hoped he will be able to further his proficiency on the hospital wards.

TABLE 1. Summary of Clinical Features of Fluid and Electrolyte Disturbances

Water Deficiency
    Loss of eyeball and skin turgor
    Dry mucous membranes
    Increased temperature and pulse
    Delirium and coma
    Concentrated urine
    Thirst
Water Excess
    Pulmonary and peripheral edema
    Abdominal and skeletal muscular twitching and
      cramps
    Stupor, coma or convulsions
Hyponatremia
    Lethargy, confusion, coma, seizures
    Muscle weakness, cramps
    Edema
    Postural hypotension
    Decreased urine output
Hypernatremia
    Lethargy, delirium, coma, convulsions
    Loss of skin turgor
    Dry mucous membranes
    Muscular weakness
    Fever, tachycardia
Hypokalemia
    Muscle weakness, cramps and paralysis
    Hyporeflexia
    Paralytic ileus
    Paresthesias, latent tetany
    Cardiac arrhythmias
    Hyposthenuria
Hyperkalemia
    Muscle weakness leading to flaccid paralysis
    Paresthesias
    Cardiac arrhythmias, heart block and cardiac standstill
Acidosis (both types)
    Hyperventilation
    Lethargy, stupor or coma
    Asterixis
    Abdominal pain
    Usually signs of dehydration (water deficiency)
Alkalosis, metabolic
    Hypoventilation
    Stupor progressing to coma
    Tetany and convulsions
    Muscle cramps
    Usually signs of hypokalemia
Alkalosis, respiratory
    Hyperventilation
    Stupor progressing to coma
    Tetany and convulsions
    Muscle cramps

TABLE 2. Typical Electrolyte Alterations in Common Clinical Disorders

Na	K	Cl	HCO$_3^-$	pH	Check Other Anions	
↑	—	↑	—	—		Dehydration—Diabetes Insipidus
↑	↓	↓	↑	↑		Primary Aldosteronism
—	—	—	↓	↓	Ketones	Starvation
—	— or ↓	↑	↓	↑	Salicylic acid	Salicylate Intoxication (early)
↓	—	↓	—	—		Pathologic Diaphoresis
↓	↓	↓	↑	↑	Ketones later	Pyloric Obstruction
↓	↓	↓	↓	↓	Ketones later	Diarrhea
↓	↑	↓	↓	— or ↓		Addison's Disease, Spironolactone Therapy
↓	↑, — or ↓	↓	↓	↓	Ketones	Diabetic Acidosis
↓	↓	↓	↑, —, ↓	↑ or —		Diuretics
↓	↑	↑	↓	— or ↓	Sulfates, Phosphates	Acute Renal Failure
↓	— or ↓	— or ↓	↓	↓	Sulfates, Phosphates	Chronic Renal Failure
— or ↓	—	↓	—	—		CHF without Diuretics
—	—	↓	↑	↓		Pulmonary Emphysema
↓	↓	—	—	—		Malabsorption Syndrome

TABLE 3. Differential Diagnosis of Single Electrolyte Changes*†

Hyponatremia
  A. Disorders of Intake and Absorption
    1. Vomiting
    2. Pyloric obstruction
    3. Diarrhea
    4. Biliary or intestinal fistula
    5. Starvation
    6. I.V. administration of 5% dextrose and water
    7. Malabsorption syndrome
  B. Disorders of Secretion
    1. Pathologic diaphoresis with replacement of water alone
    2. Burns and exudates
  C. Disorders of Excretion
    1. Diuretics
    2. Nephritis
    3. Acute and chronic renal failure
  D. Disorders of Regulation
    1. Adrenal insufficiency
    2. Cerebral salt wasting syndrome
    3. Inappropriate ADH secretion
  E. Disorders of Transport
    1. Congestive heart failure without treatment
    2. Shock
    3. Frequent paracentesis and thoracentesis
  F. Miscellaneous
    1. Advanced pulmonary disease
    2. Advanced malnutrition and cachexia
    3. Portal cirrhosis
    4. Metabolic alkalosis causing sodium to move intracellularly
    5. Diabetic acidosis
    6. Metabolic acidosis of other causes
    7. Hyperglycemia
    8. Hyperlipemia

Hypernatremia
    1. Water deprivation and dehydration
    2. Pathologic diaphoresis without water ingestion
    3. Diabetes insipidus
    4. Nephrogenic diabetes insipidus
    5. Primary aldosteronism
    6. Administration of normal saline or hypertonic saline
    7. Dehydration of prolonged coma
    8. Hypothalamic lesions with loss of thirst
    9. Tube feeding and hyperalimentation
    10. Fanconi syndrome
    11. Polyuria due to potassium depletion
    12. Hyperpnea
    13. Diarrhea, protracted
    14. Hypercalciuria
    15. Interstitial nephritis
    16. Vomiting with poor I.V. fluid replacement of water

Hypokalemia
  A. Decreased Intake
    1. Increased secretion
  B. Gastrointestinal Losses
    1. Vomiting
    2. Pyloric and other forms of intestinal obstruction
    3. Biliary or G.I. fistulas
    4. Suction
    5. Diarrhea or repeated enemas
  C. Increased Excretion
    1. Chronic renal insufficiency
    2. Potassium-losing nephritis
    3. Renal tubular acidosis
    4. Diuretics
  D. Hormonal or Regulatory Disorders
    1. Aldosteronism
    2. Cushing's syndrome
    3. Steroid therapy
    4. Diabetic acidosis
  E. Miscellaneous
    1. Acidosis of any cause
    2. Trauma or burns with tissue breakdown
    3. Intravenous administration of potassium free liquids

*Look for most striking feature of electrolyte results.
†Correlate list of possibilities in this table with clinical picture.

TABLE 3. Differential Diagnosis of Single Electrolyte Changes*† (continued)

Hyperkalemia
  A. Increased Intake or Intravenous Administration
  B. Decreased Excretion
    1. Acute renal disease
    2. Dyrenium diuretic therapy
    3. Spironolactone therapy
    4. Adrenal insufficiency
  C. Redistribution from Intracellular to Extracellular Fluid
    1. Acidosis (H^+ moves into cell, K^+ moves out)
    2. Anoxia
    3. Hyponatremia (K^+ moves out of cell to replace Na^+)、

Hypochloremia
  A. Disorders of Intake
    1. Decreased intake with normal or increased water intake
  B. Decreased Absorption
    1. Malabsorption syndrome
    2. Diarrhea
  C. Increased Secretion
    1. Pyloric and other forms of intestinal obstruction
    2. Biliary and intestinal fistulas
    3. Excessive sweating with normal water intake
    4. Vomiting
  D. Increased Excretion
    1. Chronic renal failure
    2. Diuretics
  E. Disorders of Transport
    1. Congestive heart failure
  F. Disorders of Regulation
    1. Inappropriate ADH secretion
    2. Respiratory acidosis
    3. Adrenal insufficiency
    4. Primary aldosteronism
  G. Miscellaneous
    1. Diabetic acidosis
    2. Lactic acidosis

Hyperchloremia
  A. Disorders of Intake
    1. Lack of water intake (dehydration)
    2. Ingestion of ammonium chloride
  B. Disorders of Secretion
    1. Pathologic diaphoresis without water ingestion
  C. Disorders of Excretion
    1. Renal tubular acidosis
    2. Diamox diuretics
    3. Salicylate intoxication
    4. Acute renal failure
  D. Disorders of Regulation
    1. Diabetes insipidus

Decreased Bicarbonate
  A. Disorders of Intake
    1. Starvation (leading to ketonemia)
    2. Dehydration
    3. Ingestion of acids
  B. Disorders of Secretion
    1. Diarrhea
    2. Biliary and lower intestinal fistulas
  C. Disorders of Excretion
    1. Acute and chronic renal failure
    2. Renal tubular acidosis
    3. Diuretics
    4. Salicylate intoxication
  D. Disorders of Regulation
    1. Addison's disease
  E. Miscellaneous
    1. Diabetic acidosis
    2. Lactic acidosis
    3. Specific toxin ingestion (methyl alcohol, etc.)

Increased Bicarbonate
  A. Disorders of Intake
    1. Ingestion of bicarbonate and antacids
    2. Intravenous administration of bicarbonate, lactate and citrate
  B. Disorders of Secretion
    1. Pyloric and upper intestinal obstruction
    2. Vomiting
  C. Disorders of Excretion
    1. Mercurial diuretics
    2. Pulmonary emphysema and other causes of respiratory acidosis
  D. Disorders of Regulation
    1. Primary aldosteronism

TABLE 4. Differential Diagnosis of Reported Electrolyte Results

Na	K	Cl	HCO₃⁻	Check Misc. Anions	Confirmatory Lab. Tests	Differential Diagnosis
↑	↑	↑	↑	PO₄ SO₄	Plasma protein BUN Blood gases	1. Lab. error 2. Burns with vomiting 3. Pulmonary emphysema with acute renal failure
↑	—	↑	↑		Blood gases Blood volume Hematocrit Plasma protein	1. Lab. error 2. Pulmonary emphysema and dehydration 3. Vomiting and dehydration
↑	↑	—	↑	PO₄ SO₄	Blood gases Plasma protein Hematocrit	1. Lab. error 2. Pulmonary emphysema with dehydration 3. Pyloric obstruction with renal failure
↑	↑	↑	—	PO₄ SO₄	BUN Plasma protein Blood volume	1. Second and third degree burns 2. Dehydration and renal failure 3. Lab. error
↑	↓	↑	↑		Plasma renin Blood volume	1. Lab. error 2. Dehydration 3. Aldosteronism
↑	↓	↑	—		Serum osmolality FBS	1. Lab. error 2. Hyperosmolar diabetic coma
↑	↑	↓	↑	PO₄ SO₄	Blood gases BUN Creatinine	1. Lab. error 2. Pulmonary emphysema and acute renal failure 3. Renal failure and aldosteronism
↑	↑	↑	↓	Ketones	BUN Plasma protein Blood volume	1. Burns 2. Lab. error 3. Diabetic acidosis with dehydration
↑	—	—	↑		Blood gases	1. Lab. error 2. Pyloric obstruction and dehydration 3. Pulmonary emphysema and dehydration
↑	↑	—	—	PO₄ SO₄	BUN Creatinine Plasma cortisol	1. Lab. error 2. Renal failure 3. Adrenal insufficiency
↑	—	↑	—		Blood volume Hematocrit Plasma protein Serum/urine osmolality	1. Dehydration 2. Diabetes insipidus 3. Heat stroke 4. Hyperosmolar coma
↑	—	↓	—	PO₄ SO₄	Blood volume Hematocrit Plasma protein	1. Lab. error 2. Dehydration and chronic renal failure
↑	↓	↓	↑		Plasma renin Angiography	1. Primary aldosteronism 2. Secondary aldosteronism
↑	↑	↓	↓	PO₄ SO₄	BUN & creatinine	1. Lab. error 2. Renal failure with dehydration
↑	↓	—	↓	Ketones	FBS Serum acetone	1. Lab. error 2. Diabetic acidosis 3. Potassium-losing nephritis

TABLE 4. Differential Diagnosis of Reported Electrolyte Results (Continued)

Na	K	Cl	HCO$_3^-$	Check Misc. Anions	Confirmatory Lab. Tests	Differential Diagnosis
↑	—	—	—		Plasma renin Angiography	1. Lab. error 2. Aldosteronism 3. Aldosteronism and renal failure 4. Dehydration
↑	↓	↓	↓	Ketones PO$_4$	BUN & creatinine	1. Lab. error 2. Dehydration and chronic renal failure 3. Dehydration and diabetic acidosis
—	—	↑	↑		Blood gases	1. Lab. error 2. Pulmonary emphysema and renal tubular acidosis 3. Pulmonary emphysema and diuretics
—	↑	—	↑	PO$_4$ SO$_4$	Blood gases	1. Lab. error 2. Pulmonary emphysema with renal failure 3. Pulmonary emphysema and spironolactone diuretics
—	↑	↑	—		Plasma protein BUN Plasma cortisol	1. Lab. error 2. Burns 3. Adrenal insufficiency 4. Spironolactone diuretics
—	↑	↓	↑	PO$_4$ SO$_4$	Blood gases BUN & creatinine	1. Pulmonary emphysema and renal failure 2. Pyloric obstruction and renal failure 3. Lab. error
—	↑	↑	↓	PO$_4$ SO$_4$	BUN & creatinine Urine pH	1. Acute renal failure 2. Renal tubular acidosis 3. Spironolactone diuretics
—	—	↓	↑		Blood gases BUN	1. Pulmonary emphysema 2. Pyloric obstruction, vomiting 3. Bronchial asthma 4. Milk-alkali syndrome 5. CNS—depressants
—	—	—	↑		Blood gases	1. Lab. error 2. Pyloric obstruction 3. Pulmonary emphysema
—	—	—	↓	Ketones	Blood gases Blood sugar	1. Starvation 2. Diabetic ketoacidosis 3. Shock
—	↑	—	—	PO$_4$ SO$_4$	BUN Creatinine	1. Acute renal failure 2. Spironolactone or triamterene diuretics 3. Lab. error
—	↓	↓	↑		Blood gases Plasma renin Plasma protein	1. Mercurial diuretics 2. Pulmonary emphysema 3. Aldosteronism 4. Protein-losing enteropathy
—	↑	↓	↓	PO$_4$ SO$_4$ Lactic acid Ketones	BUN Creatinine Blood volume Blood gases	1. Lab. error 2. Shock with renal failure 3. Diabetic acidosis

continued next page

TABLE 4. Differential Diagnosis of Reported Electrolyte Results (Continued)

Na	K	Cl	HCO$_3^-$	Check Misc. Anions	Confirmatory Lab. Tests	Differential Diagnosis
—	↓	↑	↓		Blood gases	1. Lab. error 2. Biliary and pancreatic fistulas 3. Renal tubular acidosis 4. Diarrhea
—	—	↑	—			1. Lab. error
—	↑	↑	↑	PO$_4$ SO$_4$	Blood volume BUN Hematocrit Plasma protein	1. Lab. error 2. Pyloric obstruction and renal failure 3. Cirrhosis of the liver
—	↓	↑	↑	PO$_4$ SO$_4$	Blood gases BUN & creatinine	1. Lab. error 2. Pulmonary emphysema and renal tubular acidosis or failure 3. Diuretics
—	—	—	—		Blood gases	1. Normal 2. Lab. error 3. Combinations of two types acidosis or two types alkalosis
—	—	↓	—		Blood volume CVP Blood gases	1. Lab. error 2. CHF 3. Pulmonary emphysema with renal tubular acidosis
—	↓	—	↓	PO$_4$ SO$_4$	BUN & creatinine	1. Chronic renal failure 2. Diuretics
—	↓	↓	↓	Ketones Lactic acid	FBS Blood volume Hematocrit Plasma proteins	1. Lab. error 2. Diabetic acidosis 3. Shock 4. Lactic acidosis
—	—	↑	↓	Ketones occas.	Blood salicylates Blood gases	1. Salicylate intoxication 2. Hyperventilation syndrome 3. Head trauma
↓	↑	↑	↑	PO$_4$ SO$_4$	BUN & creatinine pH	1. Lab. error 2. Renal failure with vomiting 3. Diuretics
↓	—	↑	↑	PO$_4$ SO$_4$	BUN & creatinine	1. Lab. error 2. Diuretics 3. Renal failure with vomiting
↓	↑	—	↑	PO$_4$ SO$_4$	BUN & creatinine	1. Acute renal failure with vomiting or intestinal obstruction
↓	↑	↑	—	PO$_4$ SO$_4$	BUN & creatinine	1. Lab. error 2. Acute renal failure 3. Spironolactone or triamterene diuretics
↓	↓	↑	↑	PO$_4$ SO$_4$	Blood gases BUN & creatinine	1. Lab. error 2. Pulmonary emphysema and renal tubular acidosis or failure 3. Diuretics

TABLE 4. Differential Diagnosis of Reported Electrolyte Results (Continued)

Na	K	Cl	HCO₃⁻	Check Misc. Anions	Confirmatory Lab. Tests	Differential Diagnosis
↓	↑	↓	↑	PO₄ SO₄	BUN & creatinine	1. Lab error 2. Pulmonary emphysema and renal failure 3. Pyloric obstruction and renal failure
↓	↑	↑	↓	PO₄ SO₄	BUN & creatinine Plasma cortisol	1. Acute renal failure 2. Adrenal insufficiency 3. Spironolactone diuretics 4. Salicylates
↓	—	↓	↓	Ketones	FBS Serum acetone	1. Diabetic acidosis 2. Diuretics
↓	—	—	↑		Blood gases	1. Pyloric obstruction 2. Pulmonary emphysema 3. Lab. error
↓	—	—	↓	PO₄ SO₄	BUN & creatinine FBS Serum acetone	1. Chronic renal failure 2. Diuretics 3. Diabetic acidosis
↓	↑	—	—	PO₄ SO₄	Plasma cortisol BUN	1. Acute renal failure 2. Adrenal insufficiency 3. Spironolactone
↓	↓	—	—		Blood gases	1. Diuretics 2. Lab. error 3. Salt-losing nephritis 4. Vomiting and diarrhea
↓	↓	↓	↑		Blood volume CVP Hematocrit Plasma proteins Blood gases	1. Pyloric obstruction 2. Pulmonary emphysema with CHF or diuretics 3. Diuretics alone
↓	↑	↓	↓	PO₄ SO₄ Ketones	Blood volume Plasma cortisol BUN & Creatinine FBS	1. Adrenal insufficiency 2. Acute renal failure 3. Spironolactone diuretics 4. Diabetic ketoacidosis
↓	—	↑	—		Plasma cortisol	1. Lab. error 2. Adrenal insufficiency 3. Diuretics
↓	—	↓	—		BUN Blood volume Hematocrit Plasma proteins CVP Serum/urine osmolality	1. Pathologic diaphoresis 2. CHF 3. Inappropriate ADH secretion 4. Acute renal failure
↓	↓	↑	↓	PO₄ SO₄	BUN Blood volume Blood gases	1. Lab. error 2. Renal tubular acidosis 3. Acetazolamide diuretic 4. Chronic renal failure
↓	↓	—	↓	PO₄ Ketones	FBS BUN & creatinine	1. Lab. error 2. Diabetic acidosis 3. Chronic renal failure

continued next page

TABLE 4. Differential Diagnosis of Reported Electrolyte Results (Continued)

Na	K	Cl	HCO₃⁻	Check Misc. Anions	Confirmatory Lab. Tests	Differential Diagnosis
↓	—	—	—		Blood gases	1. Lab. error 2. Combined acidosis or combined alkalosis
↓	↓	↓	↓	Ketones PO₄ SO₄	FBS Blood gases	1. Diarrhea 2. Diabetic acidosis 3. Renal tubular acidosis 4. Chronic renal failure 5. Diuretics
↓	↓	—	↑			1. Diuretics 2. Pyloric obstruction 3. Lab. error
↓	↓	↓	—		Serum carotene Serum/urine osmolality	1. Malabsorption syndrome 2. Diuretics 3. Inappropriate ADH syndrome 4. Pathologic diaphoresis

Note: HCO₃⁻ is HCO_3^-; PO₄ is PO_4; SO₄ is SO_4.

TABLE 5. Differential Diagnosis of Blood Gas Disturbances

PO_2	P_{CO_2}	pH	HCO_3^-	Differential Diagnosis
↓	—	—	—	1. CHF 2. Pulmonary embolism 3. Sarcoidosis 4. Pulmonary fibrosis 5. V-A shunt
↓	↓	↑	↓	1. Early status asthmaticus 2. Adult respiratory distress syndrome 3. Shock of several causes—early 4. Pulmonary embolism
↓	↑	↓	↑	1. Pulmonary emphysema—late 2. Barbiturate intoxication 3. Poliomyelitis and other CNS disorders 4. Late status asthmaticus
—	↓	↑	↓	1. Salicylate intoxication 2. Hyperventilation syndrome
—	↑	—	↑	1. Early pulmonary emphysema (compensated respiratory acidosis) 2. Compensated metabolic alkalosis
—	↓	↓	↓	1. Diabetic acidosis 2. Other forms of metabolic acidosis 3. Shock—late stages with adequate O_2 therapy
↑	↓	↑	↑	1. Overuse of IPPB in pulmonary emphysema
—	↓	—	↓	1. High altitude living (compensated respiratory alkalosis)

Section Four

Clinical Disorders of
Fluid and Electrolyte Balance

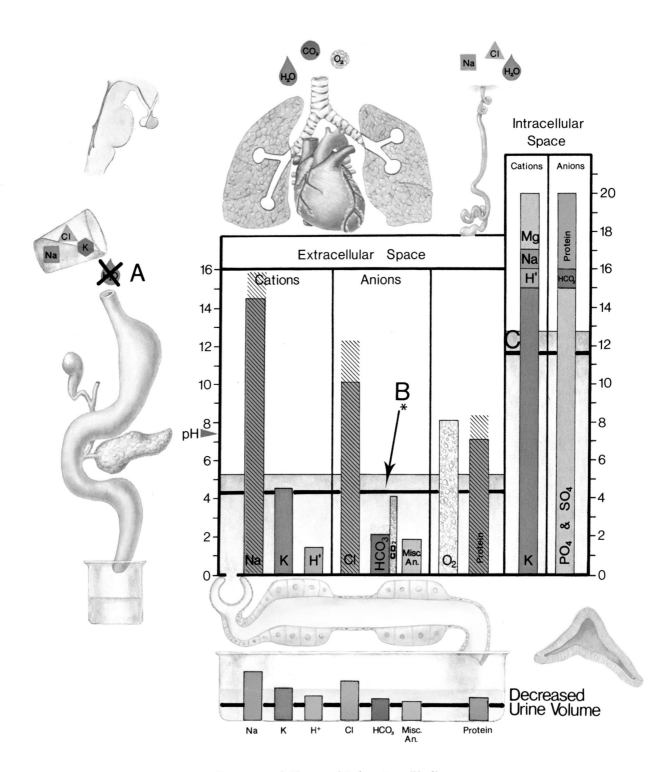

Summary of Abnormal Laboratory Findings

Serum Na—increased
Serum K—normal
Serum Cl—increased
Serum HCO_3^-—normal
  or decreased

Serum protein—
  increased
Blood volume—
  decreased*
Urine volume—
  decreased

Dehydration

Pathophysiology

Typically a decreased ingestion of water (A) leads to a decrease in plasma volume (B), as well as extracellular and intracellular volume (C) because the obligatory loss of water through the skin, lung and kidney continues. Blood levels of *sodium* and *chloride* increase markedly both because of hemoconcentration and the enhancement of tubular reabsorption of these electrolytes by the stimulus of a contracted circulatory volume on the osmoreceptor-aldosterone system. Since at least 40 mEq. of *potassium* continues to be lost each day, its level does not rise unless there is associated acute renal failure. The HCO_3^- level does not alter unless there is associated starvation or other acid-base disorder. Urine volume drops and the specific gravity and osmolality rise if kidney function and ADH action are good.

Clinical Picture

The eyeballs are mushy, the skin tents, the mucous membranes are dry and the urine is a deep yellow or orange. There may be confusion, muscular weakness and signs of an underlying illness (cerebrovascular disease) which caused the dehydration.

Diagnosis

There is frequently no history, but if the patient has been hospitalized for some time a look at the nurses' notes or an intake and output sheet may be helpful. Weighing the patient will show a change if the weight prior to illness is known. Serum electrolytes will show the marked elevation of *sodium* and *chloride*. A rise in hematocrit and *protein* will often confirm this, but since many of these patients suffer from malnutrition and anemia this may be helpful only if previous values are known. Blood volume, if performed accurately, will be of more help. The BUN may rise, usually without much rise in the creatinine. Finally the urine specific gravity and osmolality are very high.

Treatment

Initially 5 per cent dextrose and water is administered according to the water deficit calculated with the following formula:

$$\text{Deficit of water} = \frac{\text{Normal sodium concentration}}{\text{Present sodium concentration}} \times \text{Normal body water}$$

OR

$$\text{Deficit of water} = \frac{138}{\text{Present sodium concentration}} \times 60\% \text{ of body weight in Kg.}$$

The fluid must not be administered too rapidly because the glucose will induce a solute diuresis[8] and prevent adequate replacement. Furthermore, potassium and often sodium must be given once volume expansion takes place. The necessity for these electrolytes will be evidenced by serum electrolyte determinations every two to four hours initially.

Etiology

The picture described here is one of pure dehydration which does not often occur alone. There may be a loss of sodium in excess of water or an isotonic loss of sodium and water. The serum sodium and chloride therefore may be normal or low in some circumstances with a contracted circulatory volume.

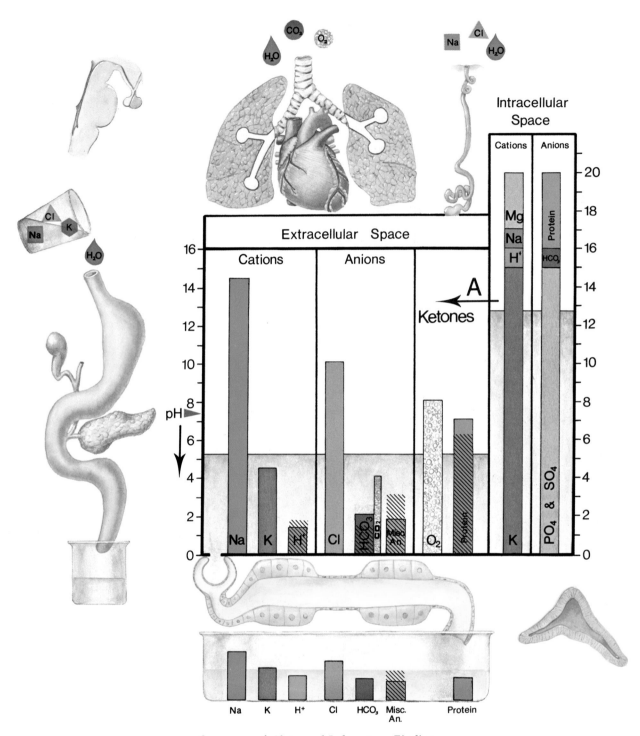

Summary of Abnormal Laboratory Findings

Serum K—normal or
   increased
Serum H⁺—increased
   or normal
Serum HCO₃⁻—
   decreased
Serum miscellaneous
   anions—increased

Serum protein—
   decreased
Blood pH—decreased
   or normal
Blood volume—
   decreased or normal
Urine volume—
   decreased or normal

Starvation

Pathogenesis

Lack of food ingestion, either primary or secondary to anorexia nervosa and various neurologic or upper gastrointestinal disorders, causes fat and protein to be catabolized for energy. Various organic acids are produced in this fashion including *ketones* (A). As in diabetic acidosis the supply of keto-acids exceeds the demands of the cells and their plasma levels *rise* (miscellaneous anions). Plasma bicarbonate decreases, since it is utilized in neutralizing these acids. However, the by-product, carbon dioxide, is blown off by the lungs so that the resulting metabolic acid is well compensated for and the *pH* drops very little.

Clinical Picture

Extreme emaciation and muscle wasting is evident and there may be edema of the lower extremities, although this is not of cardiac origin. Pulse is often rapid, the blood pressure low and signs of dehydration (page 77) may be present. Other objective findings are those of the underlying disorder (senile dementia, cerebral arteriosclerosis, etc.).

Diagnosis

In addition to the electrolyte changes mentioned above blood and urine acetone and urea are usually elevated.

Treatment

These individuals respond to small frequent feedings surprisingly well, although the cardiovascular system may take months to return to normal.

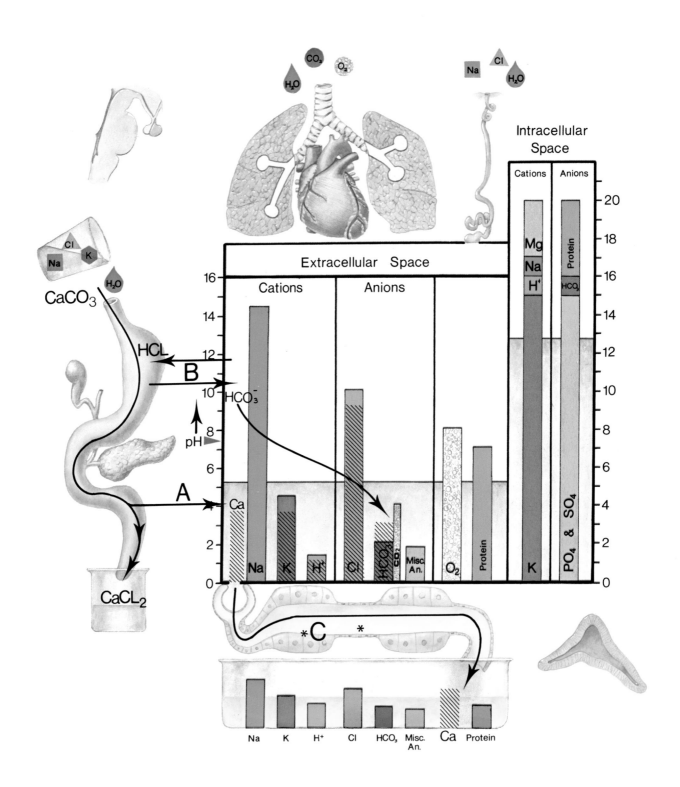

Summary of Abnormal Laboratory Findings

Serum K—decreased	Blood pH—increased
Serum H⁺—decreased	Serum and urine
Serum HCO₃⁻—	Ca—increased
increased	Ca deposits in kidney*
Serum Cl—decreased	

Milk-Alkali Syndrome

Pathophysiology

The ingestion of large amounts of nonabsorbable antacids such as calcium carbonate with or without milk neutralizes HCl in the gastric juice by the following equation:

$$CaCO_3 + 2HCl \longrightarrow CaCl_2 + H_2CO_3$$

The weak acid H_2CO_3 dissipates and much of the $CaCl_2$ passes into the stool. However some is absorbed, creating *hypercalcemia* (A). The neutralization of the HCl stimulates further secretion of HCl and bicarbonate is released into the serum (B) as a by-product. Thus *serum bicarbonate rises* and a metabolic alkalosis ensues. This may precipitate deposits of calcium in the kidney (C) and other tissues. The chloride secreted in the gastric juice is not adequately reabsorbed as calcium chloride and *serum chloride drops*. The metabolic alkalosis precipitates a *drop in serum potassium* by the methods discussed on page 45. If sodium bicarbonate were the antacid employed, a similar turn of events would follow, but in addition some of the sodium bicarbonate would be absorbed and aggravate the alkalosis further.

Clinical Picture

Symptoms and signs of tetany such as muscular twitching, cramping, carpopedal spasms and convulsions are the usual findings, because even though the serum calcium is usually elevated there may be less in an ionized form. Symptoms of renal stones and azotemia may develop.

Diagnosis

Hypercalcemia, hypercalciuria, increased serum bicarbonate and pH in patients with ulcer disease and a history of ingestion of antacids and milk are the most significant diagnostic features. BUN and creatinine may be elevated and a flat plate of the abdomen may show nephrocalcinosis or renal stones.

Treatment

The antacids are stopped. The chloride and potassium deficits may be calculated and replaced fairly quickly with hypotonic saline and potassium chloride if renal function is adequate. Otherwise treatment must be more cautious.

Etiology

The ingestion of a wide variety of antacids (magnesium hydroxide, magnesium trisilicate, etc.) may induce this picture, but sodium bicarbonate is the worst offender.

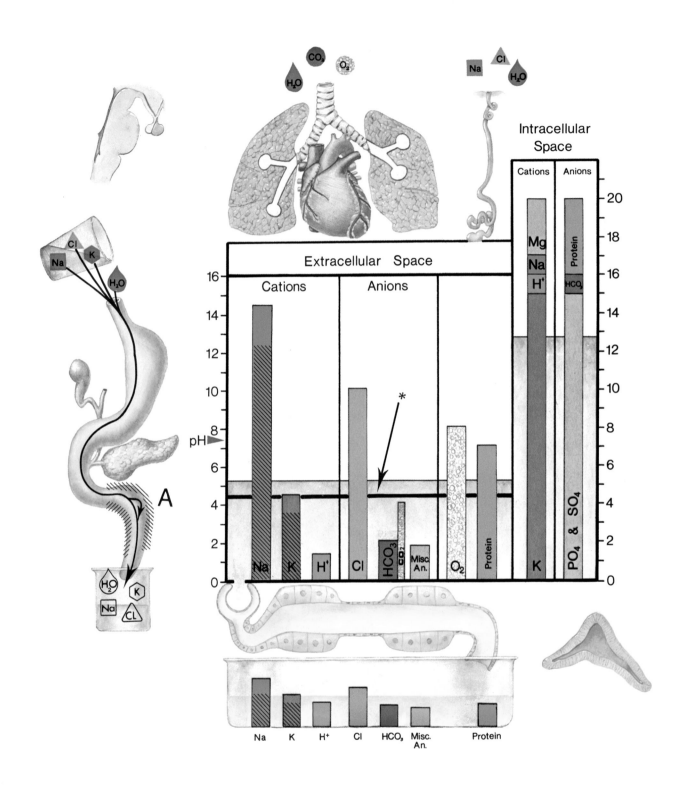

Summary of Abnormal Laboratory Findings
Serum Na—decreased
Serum K—decreased
Blood volume—
    decreased*
Urine Na—decreased
Urine K—decreased

Malabsorption Syndrome

Pathophysiology

The poor absorption of water and salts in this disorder (A) leads to *hyponatremia, hypokalemia* and a *drop in circulatory* and *intracellular volume*. This occurs primarily in advanced cases in which there is significant loss of mucosal surface or infiltration by inflammatory or proteinaceous elements.

Clinical Picture

This will resemble a combination of starvation (page 79) and dehydration (page 77). There will be bloating and abdominal distention along with diarrhea in most cases. If there is an associated malabsorption of calcium there may be compression and Milkman's fractures. Emotional disturbances are common.

Diagnosis

Good screening tests for this disorder are the D-xylose absorption test, the serum carotene and urine for 5-HIAA (5-hydroxyindoleacetic acid). However, a mucosal biopsy is best for establishing the diagnosis.

Treatment

In nontropical sprue the response to a gluten-free diet is both diagnostic and therapeutic. Treatment with antibiotics may be effective in cases of blind loop syndrome, scleroderma, Whipple's disease, etc. where there is bacterial overgrowth. Steroids are useful in regional enteritis and hypogammaglobulinemia. A low fat diet is useful in intestinal lymphangiectasia. An increased oral intake of water, salt and potassium may restore proper electrolyte balance in some cases, but intravenous therapy should be resorted to in acute cases. The sodium and potassium deficits may be calculated using the formulas on page 156.

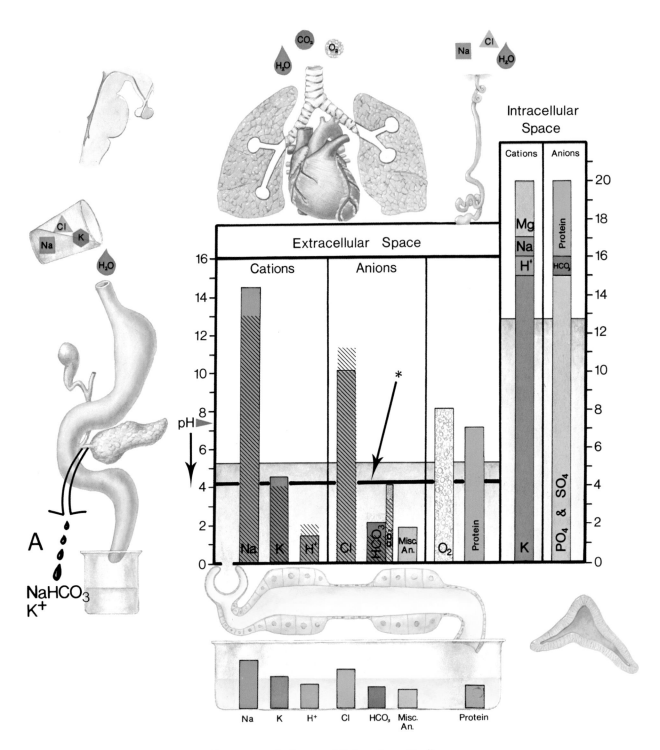

Summary of Abnormal Laboratory Findings

Serum Na—normal or
    decreased
Serum H⁺—increased
Serum K—decreased or
    normal
Serum HCO₃⁻—
    decreased

Serum Cl—increased or
    normal
Blood pH—decreased
Blood Pco₂—decreased
Blood volume—
    decreased*

Biliary and Pancreatic Fistulas

Pathophysiology

These result from postoperative complications as a rule. Up to a liter of alkaline fluid containing large amounts of sodium (120 mEq./L.) and bicarbonate (60-150 mEq./L.) may be lost each day, particularly in pancreatic fistulas (A). This leads to a metabolic acidosis with a *drop* in serum bicarbonate and blood pH and P_{CO_2} and a compensatory *rise in serum chloride* to try to maintain anion balance. *Serum hydrogen ion* usually rises as a by-product of bicarbonate production by the pancreas. Serum sodium is lost, but its concentration may remain the same since *blood volume* may drop concomitantly. Although bile and pancreatic juice contain less potassium than gastric juice (3-12 mEq./L.), the serum potassium may drop if this is not replaced for several days. Because of fat, protein and carbohydrate breakdown and poor absorption, severe weight loss and malnutrition may develop.

Clinical Picture

There may be hyperventilation, dehydration, clouded sensorium and signs of hypokalemia (page 39) and malabsorption syndrome (page 83). The malnutrition may lead to poor wound healing.

Diagnosis

In most cases the diagnosis will be obvious clinically unless the fistula drains into the colon. The changes in serum electrolytes and blood pH will support the diagnosis.

Treatment

This is primarily directed at correction of the fistula. Until that is accomplished fluid and electrolytes in the amount lost are replaced. Some physicians simply put these back through a nasogastric tube. Lactated potassic saline solution (Darrow's) may be used in amounts equaling the losses. However, this and Isolyte E with 5 percent dextrose will provide more chloride than necessary (103 or 111 mEq./L.). It is better to use half normal saline with one ampule of sodium bicarbonate (44.6 mEq.) and 10 to 20 mEq. of KCl added.

Etiology

This has already been discussed above.

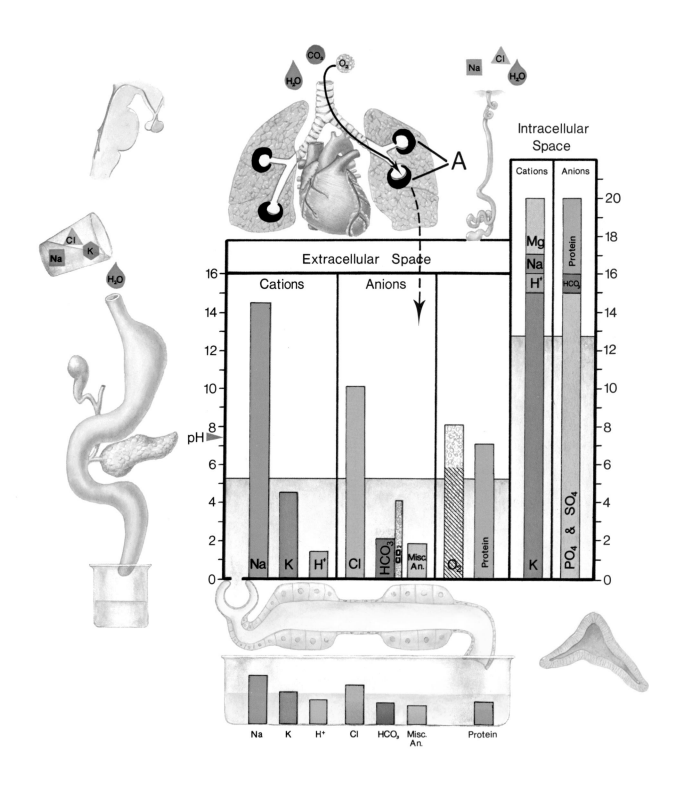

Summary of Abnormal Laboratory Findings
Arterial blood Po₂—decreased

Sarcoidosis

Pathophysiology

The chronic granulomatous process in this disorder thickens the alveolar-capillary membranes (A) and causes a block in oxygen absorption. This is in effect a "malabsorption syndrome" of the lung. *Blood P_{O_2} drops* but P_{CO_2} and pH do not change because carbon dioxide has a much greater solubility and diffusion capacity. Electrolyte and acid-base balance are not disturbed unless there are other disease processes involved.

Clinical Picture

There may be cyanosis, clubbing and other signs of chronic anoxia. Involvement of other organ systems (skin, nervous system) may be seen.

Diagnosis

The findings of a low arterial blood P_{O_2} with normal P_{CO_2} and pH are significant. This may only be found after exercise in early cases. Roentgenograms of the chest and hands, a positive Kveim test and scalene node biopsy will confirm the diagnosis. Pulmonary function tests may show a decreased vital capacity with a normal timed vital capacity.

Treatment

Corticosteroids may halt the progress of this disease and oxygen therapy may be necessary in late stages.

Etiology

The etiology of sarcoidosis remains unknown. The Hamman-Rich syndrome, miliary tuberculosis, anthracosilicosis, scleroderma and beryllium poisoning may produce a similar picture.

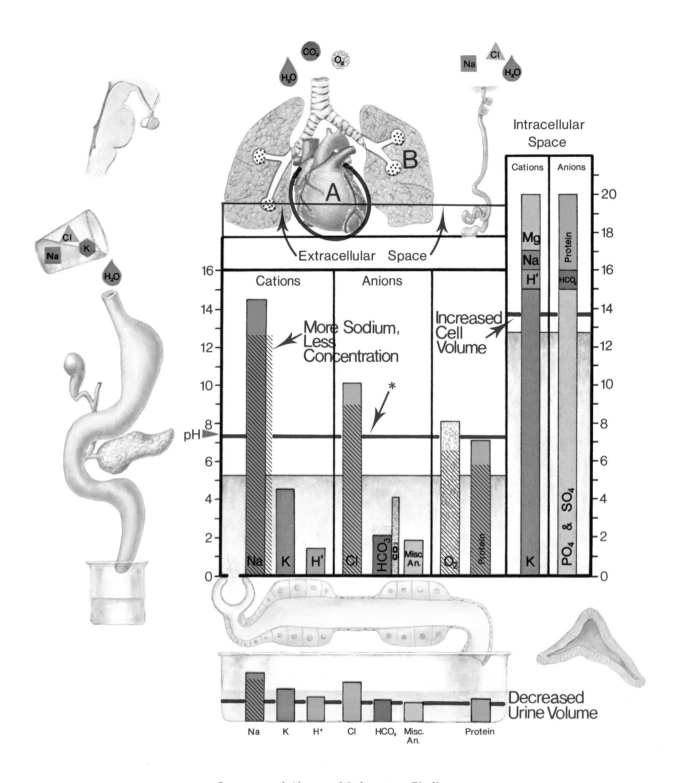

Summary of Abnormal Laboratory Findings

Serum Na—normal or   Blood volume—
  decreased   increased*
Serum Cl—normal or   Urine Na—decreased or
  decreased   normal
Serum protein—   Urine volume—
  decreased   decreased.

Congestive Heart Failure—Severe

Pathophysiology

Circulatory insufficiency in this disorder leads to retention of sodium and water by the kidney and an increase in *plasma, extracellular* and *intracellular volume*. The serum concentration of sodium will vary in proportion to the amounts of water retained with the sodium, but it is usually normal. However, in severe cases of failure more water will be retained and *dilutional hyponatremia* may develop as shown in the diagram. The exact mechanism of sodium and water retention is still disputed. According to the "backward failure theory," the failure in the "pump" leads to damming up of blood in the venous system and an increase in venous pressure and consequently impedes the movement of interstitial fluid back into the capillaries, resulting in edema. According to the "forward failure theory" a decrease in cardiac output results in a decreased glomerular filtration and increase in tubular reabsorption of sodium and water. Part of this reabsorption could be due to "secondary aldosteronism." The decreased renal blood flow stimulates the juxtaglomerular apparatus to secrete renin which activates the angiotensin system and subsequently stimulates aldosterone secretion from the adrenal cortex and enhances tubular sodium reabsorption. The temporary increase in sodium may in turn activate the osmoreceptors of the supraoptic nucleus to secrete ADH and promote water retention as well. Continuation of this vicious cycle would account for the eventual dilutional hyponatremia.

Clinical Picture

There is usually cardiomegaly (A), pulmonary edema (B), hepatomegaly, neck vein distention and pretibial or presacral edema. In pure "right-sided failure" the lungs are usually clear. *Urine volume* will be *decreased* and the specific gravity and osmolality increased, unless diuretics are being given or there is concomitant renal disease.

Diagnosis

The venous pressure will usually be elevated while the arm-to-tongue circulation time (using sodium dehydrocholate or calcium gluconate) will be prolonged (above 15 seconds). In pure left heart failure the venous pressure may be normal, but pulmonary capillary wedge pressure (measured with a Swan-Gantz catheter) will be elevated. *Arterial oxygen content* will be reduced without a change in pH or rise in P_{CO_2}. Vital capacity will be reduced without a concomitant reduction in timed vital capacity in left heart failure. A blood volume study may be useful in borderline cases. It will invariably be elevated unless there is absolute hypoproteinemia. Hematocrit and *serum protein* will be *decreased* by the dilutional effect of the large circulatory volume. All of these studies will help differentiate the dilutional hyponatremia from absolute hyponatremia occurring in cases of metabolic acidosis, after prolonged diuretic therapy and chronic renal disease.

Treatment

In addition to digitalis and diuretics, both sodium and water restriction must be resorted to when the failure is this severe. Administration of hypertonic saline solutions will only aggravate the condition and have no place in therapy. One should always look for the cause of the congestive failure, since this may be treatable (hypothyroidism, etc.)

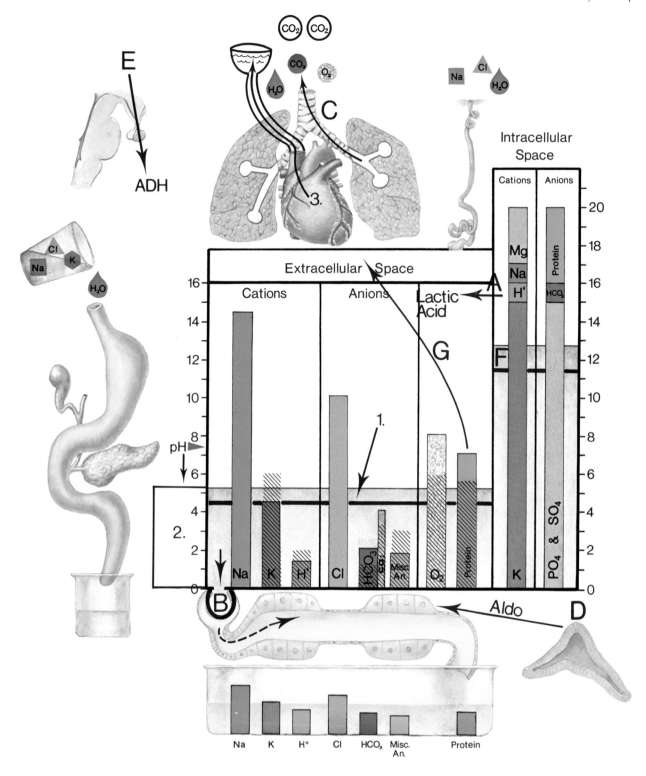

Summary of Abnormal Laboratory Findings

Serum K—increased

Serum H⁺—increased

Serum HCO₃⁻—
  decreased

Serum miscellaneous
  anions—increased

Blood volume—
  decreased

Blood Po₂—decreased

Blood Pco₂—decreased

Blood pH—decreased

Plasma protein—
  decreased usually

Shock

Pathophysiology

Shock may be due to an absolute decrease in circulatory volume (1.) (hemorrhage, hypoproteinemia, dehydration or hyponatremia) a relative decrease in circulatory volume (2.) (due to an increase in the circulatory compartment) as in neurogenic shock, or a shift of the volume to the venous side of the circulation so that the effective circulatory volume is diminished as in cardiogenic shock (3.). Whatever the cause the following metabolic, fluid and electrolyte changes take place: the *blood* P_{O_2} *drops* because of poor lung perfusion. Decreased tissue perfusion contributes to the tissue hypoxia and there is a decrease in conversion of lactate to pyruvate so that a lactic acidosis (A) may develop *increasing* the *miscellaneous anions* and *hydrogen ion* values and *decreasing bicarbonate*. Increased tissue catabolism of protein and fat releases ketones, phosphates and sulfates into the blood further increasing the *miscellaneous anions* and aggravating the metabolic acidosis. Decreased perfusion of the kidneys (B) leads to *retention of potassium, decreased excretion* of *miscellaneous anions* (phosphates, etc.) and decreased formation of bicarbonate and further aggravation of the metabolic acidosis. The lung compensates by blowing off more carbon dioxide (C). The drop in circulatory volume and the decreased renal perfusion activate the renin-angiotensin system to release aldosterone from the adrenal cortex (D) causing sodium retention, and the consequent increase in serum osmolality activates the hypothalamus (E) to secrete ADH and cause water retention. Thus there is usually no net change in serum sodium or chloride. Nevertheless, these compensatory mechanisms may be inadequate in severe shock so that the *intracellular fluid volume drops* (F) as it is transferred extracellularly. Tissue anoxia leads to increased capillary permeability and protein leaks into the extracellular space (G). Therefore *plasma protein drops.*

Clinical Picture

A cold sweat, cyanosis, and rapid pulse may precede the actual drop in blood pressure (which signifies at least a 25 per cent absolute or relative drop in circulatory volume). The pressure may rise after an initial drop due to the release of catecholamines and hydrocortisone. The patient becomes delirious, may lapse into coma and there is hyperventilation to compensate for the metabolic acidosis. Oliguria and anuria are common. Reflex nausea and vomiting occur.

Diagnosis

The clinical picture usually establishes the diagnosis, and serum electrolytes and blood gases merely confirm it. The cause may not be apparent clinically (internal bleeding, pulmonary embolism, etc.) and must be confirmed by other methods (CBC, EKG, lung scan, blood volume, etc.).

Treatment

Whatever the cause, the most important measure is to increase the circulatory volume and tissue perfusion. This will be done primarily with blood in hemorrhagic shock, but in the other forms the volume is increased using one-fourth blood, one-fourth plasma and one-half balanced electrolyte solutions (Table 6). Up to four liters of fluid often are given in the first four to six hours, but careful monitoring of central venous pressure must accompany the rapid administration of fluid. Oxygen by nose is given to correct the tissue hypoxia and lactic acidosis. Since there is already a high level of circulating catecholamines, vasopressors are no longer commonly resorted to in most cases of shock. However, steroids are given in large doses (equivalent of 500-2,000 mg. of hydrocortisone every six hours) to potentiate the effects of catecholamines and inhibit the effects of histamine and various vasoactive peptides. To improve tissue perfusion, vasodilators that also stimulate cardiac output (such as Isuprel and Dopamine) may be used.[13] The main object of therapy is not to bring the blood pressure back to normal, but to establish normal urine output. In this way the acidosis and hyperkalemia can be brought under control. In cardiogenic shock digitalis may be used with caution. Isuprel must be given more carefully in cases of myocardial infarction, because it may produce dangerous arrhythmias.

Etiology

This has been discussed under "pathophysiology." For a more detailed discussion one is referred to standard medical textbooks.[13,14]

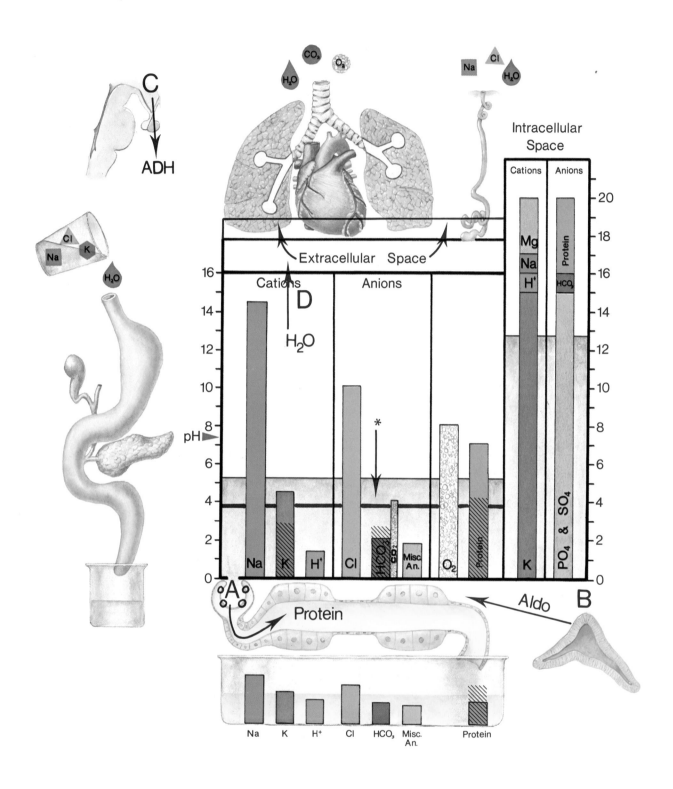

Summary of Abnormal Laboratory Findings

Serum K—decreased or normal

Serum HCO_3^-—increased or normal

Blood volume—decreased*

Serum protein—decreased

Urine protein—increased

Nephrotic Syndrome

Pathophysiology

Increased permeability of the glomerular capillary basement membrane (A) leads to leakage of plasma protein into the glomerular filtrate and urine. *Plasma protein drops* while *urine protein increases* The hypoproteinemia causes a *drop* in *circulatory volume*. This leads to a decreased renal perfusion and activation of the renin-angiotensin system with subsequent release of aldosterone (B). Sodium is retained, but the temporary hyperosmolality induces ADH secretion from the hypothalamus and pituitary (C). Thus while total body sodium and water increase, serum sodium does not usually change because the increased fluid goes into the extracellular space, causing edema (D). The secondary aldosteronism may cause an *increased bicarbonate,* alkalosis and *decreased potassium* (see page 125).

Clinical Picture

The most striking features are pitting edema and generalized anasarca.

Diagnosis

This is established by hypoproteinemia, hypercholesterolemia and a typical protein electrophoretic pattern and marked proteinuria (sometimes 3.5 gm. a day).[13] In contrast to congestive heart failure, blood volume is low. The exact cause is determined by renal biopsy and other laboratory data (antinuclear antibody test). Blood urea nitrogen and creatinine are usually normal or only slightly elevated.

Treatment

The patient should be placed on a high protein diet (100-150 gm. a day) unless significant uremia is present. Mild diuretics such as a thiazide combined with spironolactone may combat the edema and secondary hyperaldosteronism, but these should not be used too vigorously since the patient is already hypovolemic. Occasionally stronger diuretics (furosemide, etc.) are necessary. The infusion of salt-poor albumin may be useful in emergencies to increase circulatory volume. Depending on the etiology, corticosteroid therapy may be used especially in cases due to subacute glomerulonephritis and collagen disease.

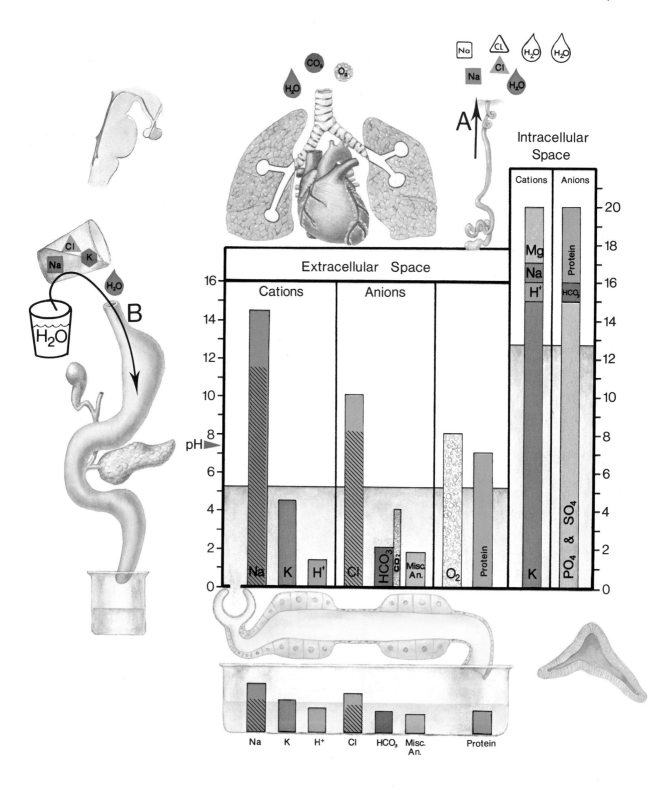

Summary of Abnormal Laboratory Findings

Serum Na—decreased	Urine Cl—decreased
Serum Cl—decreased	Urine volume—normal
Urine Na—decreased	or increased

Pathologic Diaphoresis

Pathophysiology

Excessive sweating, such as that which occurs in people in environments with high temperature or during fever, leads to a marked loss of water and moderate losses of sodium and chloride (A) (30-45 mEq./L.). As long as the oral intake of water is not restricted (B), the *serum* concentration of *sodium* and *chloride* excretion will be *decreased* to a minimum.

Clinical Picture

Symptoms usually do not occur until the serum sodium drops below 115 mEq./L. There may be abdominal and skeletal muscle cramps, nausea, weakness and confusion and occasional convulsions and coma.

Diagnosis

To differentiate this form of hyponatremia from salt-wasting nephritis and adrenal insufficiency a spot urine sodium can be done. In pathologic diaphoresis this will show a sodium of 10 mEq./L. or less. Dilutional hyponatremia can be distinguished by a high blood volume and low plasma protein, neither of which occur in this disorder.

Treatment

The sodium deficit is calculated on the basis of the following formula:

$$\text{Sodium deficit} = \text{ideal serum sodium} - \text{measured serum sodium} \times .20 \times \text{body weight in Kg.}$$

The deficit is overcome by administration of normal or hypertonic saline according to the urgency of the clinical situation. In general it is not wise to change the serum sodium more than 10 mEq. in a 24-hour period.[4] Hypertonic saline should not be administered faster than 1-2 ml./min.

Etiology

As discussed under pathophysiology.

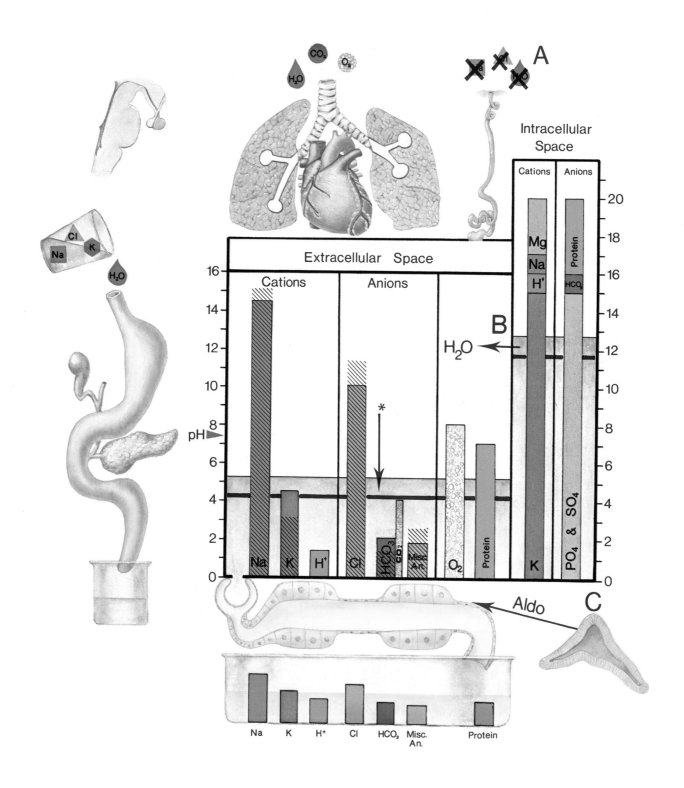

Summary of Abnormal Laboratory Findings
Serum Na—increased   Serum HCO₃⁻—
   or normal   decreased or normal
Serum K—decreased or   Blood volume—
   normal   decreased*
Serum Cl—increased or
   normal

Heat Stroke

Pathophysiology

In this disorder prolonged sweating may at first cause severe water and moderate salt depletion as seen in pathologic diaphoresis. The *plasma* and *extracellular volume* are *decreased*. Then due to continued exposure to a hot humid environment and often moderate to strenuous exercise, sweating comes to a halt (A). The exact cause of the anhidrosis is unknown, but may be disturbance of the thermoregulatory center, early shock or overworked sweat glands. Although most of these patients at this point have an *increased serum sodium and chloride*, these values may be normal because of the shifting of fluid out of the cells (B). Cessation of sweating also leads to a temperature rise and shock worsens. Tissue hypoxia develops leading to lactic acidosis with a *drop in serum bicarbonate*. The low plasma volume activates the renin-angiotensin-aldosterone system (C) to conserve salt at the expense of potassium. Consequently at least half of these patients may have a *low serum potassium*.

Clinical Picture

Hyperpyrexia (temperatures of 106°F. and above), shock without sweating, delirium, coma and even convulsions are the usual findings. Most patients get little warning, but there may be headache, weakness and dizziness. There is usually hyperventilation from the metabolic acidosis. In later stages due to DIC there may be petechiae and hemorrhages from various body orifices.

Diagnosis

The history of heat exposure and the clinical picture combined with a normal spinal fluid and the serum electrolyte changes mentioned above usually establish the diagnosis and rule out meningitis and other causes of severe hyperpyrexia. A high BUN and some elevation of the creatinine may be noted.

Treatment

Rapid reduction in body temperature with an ice water bath is the most important therapeutic measure (a hypothermic blanket may be used). The bath should be discontinued when the patient's temperature reaches 102°F. because a further drop usually occurs spontaneously. Plasma and extracellular fluid volume is replaced with 5 percent dextrose and water and half normal saline after calculating the water deficit using the formula on page 156. The potassium deficit is also calculated according to the formula on page 156 and it is treated with the 5 percent dextrose and water and half normal saline as 20 to 40 mEq. for each 1,000 ml. of fluid. Since severe lactic acidosis is not common, bicarbonate is needed only occasionally. Again the deficit is calculated with the formula on page 156 and only enough to make up half the deficit is given before a reassessment is made.

Etiology

Maxwell and Kleeman[2] have provided an extensive discussion of this, but three factors seem to be most important: (1) Prolonged exposure to a high temperature in which only evaporation of sweat can provide heat loss from the body and this is crippled by a high humidity. (2) Prolonged moderate to strenuous exercise in environments with moderate to severe elevations in temperature and humidity. (3) Predisposing factors such as arteriosclerosis, diabetes mellitus and alcoholism.

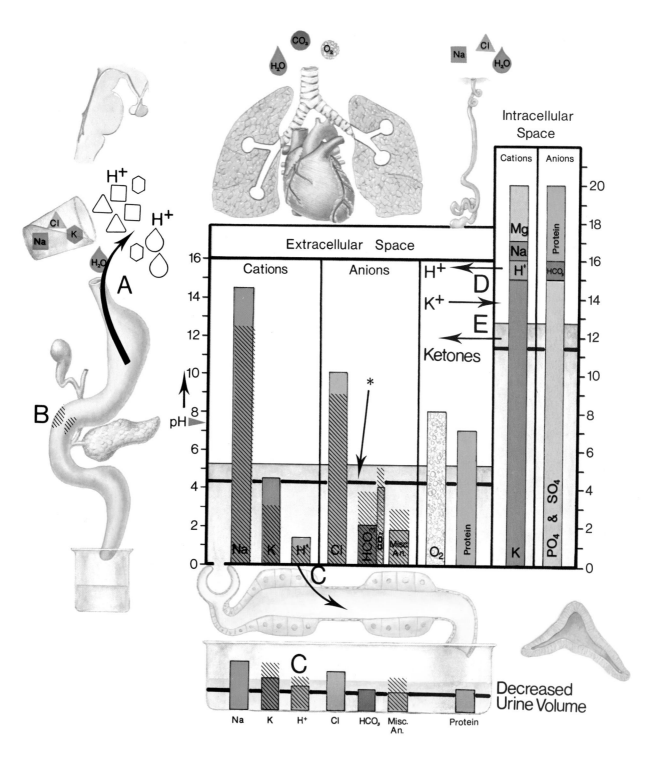

Summary of Abnormal Laboratory Findings

Serum Na—decreased
or normal
Serum K—decreased
Serum Cl—decreased
Serum HCO₃⁻—
increased

Serum H⁺—decreased
Blood pH—increased
Blood volume—
decreased*
Urine K—increased or
normal

Urine pH—decreased
or normal
Urine volume—
decreased
Urine HCO₃⁻—
increased or normal

Pyloric Obstruction

Pathophysiology

In this condition large amounts of gastric secretions containing *water, hydrogen ion, potassium, sodium and chloride are lost* orally (A) with a consequent drop in their blood levels and in *blood volume*. The constricted pylorus (B) prevents the passage of gastric juice into the intestines where it is absorbed under normal conditions. Instead it accumulates in the stomach and is vomited or must be removed by nasogastric suction. A by-product of gastric secretion of hydrochloric acid, *bicarbonate accumulates in the blood* resulting in a metabolic alkalosis. This alkalosis is further aggravated by the low serum chloride that forces the kidney to reabsorb sodium with bicarbonate.

Compensatory mechanisms (also discussed and illustrated on page 61 on compensated metabolic alkalosis) are brought into play. Respirations decrease resulting in *carbon dioxide retention* and carbonic acid production to balance the alkalosis. There is accelerated renal excretion of *sodium and potassium bicarbonate* and their levels *rise* in the *urine*. However the potassium deficit tends to diminish the exchange of potassium for sodium reabsorption in the renal tubule and *hydrogen ion* is exchanged instead. This may cause a paradoxical aciduria (C). Serum potassium is further reduced by its movement into the cell (D) to bring hydrogen ion out. Later the reduced intake of carbohydrate and other nutrients lead to fat and protein catabolism with ketosis (E) and a rise in BUN. To compensate for the drop in circulatory volume intracellular fluid and electrolytes move extracellularly and the *intracellular fluid volume drops*.

Clinical Picture

There is recurrent vomiting, often projectile in nature, associated with postprandial fullness and a vague aching pain which is relieved by the vomiting. There are signs of dehydration (page 77), respirations are often depressed and the urine output is decreased. Large peristaltic waves and a mass (the hypertrophied pylorus) may be found in the upper abdomen.

Diagnosis

An upper gastrointestinal series will show the huge dilated stomach and the gastric outlet obstruction, but usually will not reveal the exact pathology until the stomach is decompressed. In severe cases it is better to resort to gastroscopy immediately. This may show a duodenal or pyloric ulcer, carcinoma of the stomach, pancreatic pseudocyst or various other lesions. In infants the diagnosis is best established by an exploratory laparotomy.

Treatment

After establishing effective nasogastric suction, it is usually wise to restore the fluid and electrolytes to normal before proceeding with surgery or other definitive treatment. The replacement fluids must contain adequate sodium, chloride and potassium. Isotonic saline with potassium chloride added is the mainstay of treatment. Occasionally water loss is greater than salt loss and hypotonic saline must be used. Chloride, water and potassium losses are calculated using the formulas on page 156. Enough to make up half of these losses is given and the electrolytes rechecked before giving the rest. Daily losses from nasogastric suction must be replaced according to the volume and expected concentration of electrolytes in gastric juice (page 158). Daily maintenance requirements (page 157) must be given in addition to these losses and there must be careful monitoring of urine output. Occasionally gastric decompression may "cure" the obstruction (caused by significant edema in such cases) in 72 hours. If not, surgery should not be delayed beyond 92 hours.[14]

Etiology

This is usually due to a duodenal or pyloric ulcer or carcinoma in adults. Pyloric spasm and pyloric stenosis are seen in infants. The same picture may result from prolonged vomiting regardless of the cause, prolonged gastric suction, gastrocolic fistulas and the chronic ingestion of antacids in large amounts.

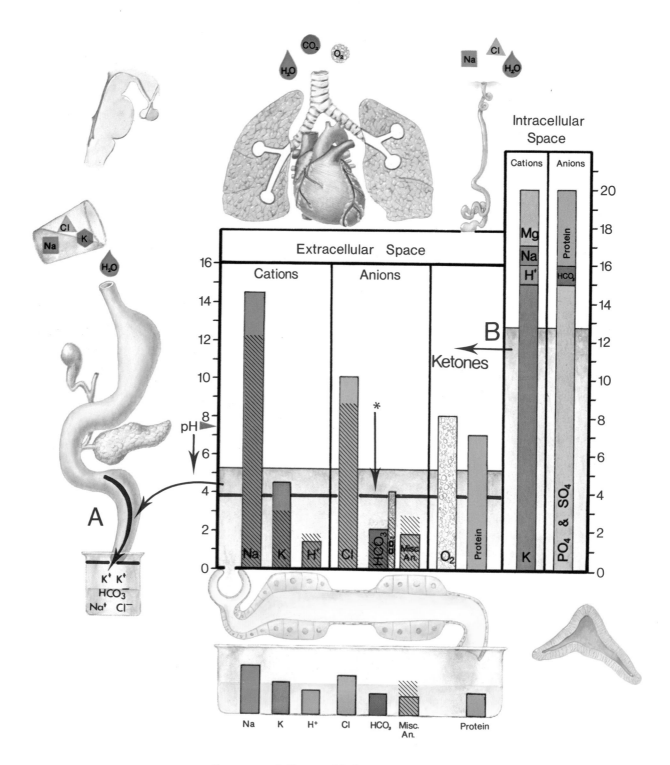

Summary of Abnormal Laboratory Findings

Serum Na—decreased
Serum K—decreased
Serum H⁺—increased
Serum Cl—decreased
Serum HCO₃⁻—
    decreased

Serum miscellaneous
    anions—increased or
    normal
Blood volume—
    decreased*
Blood pH—decreased

Diarrhea

Pathophysiology

Whether due to secretory diarrhea (as in cholera) or exudative diarrhea (as in salmonellosis, shigellosis and ulcerative colitis) large amounts of water (as much as 10 liters a day), sodium (up to 350 mEq./L.), potassium (up to 45 mEq./L.) bicarbonate and chloride are lost in the stool (A). *Circulatory volume drops.* The blood levels of *sodium, potassium, chloride and bicarbonate* all *decrease,* but since the intestinal juices contain more bicarbonate than chloride this anion diminishes to a greater extent and a metabolic acidosis develops. In cholera more chloride is lost (80-100 mEq./L.). Ketonemia, (B) produced by the lack of carbohydrate ingestion, *increases* the serum *miscellaneous anions* and aggravates the acidosis. In severe cases shock develops, reducing the compensatory action of the kidney and further aggravating the acidosis. *Hydrogen ion increases* and the pH drops. In exudative diarrhea there may be protein loss (see page 103).

Clinical Picture

There is diarrhea, signs of dehydration (page 77), hyperventilation to compensate for the metabolic acidosis, oliguria, shock and sometimes delirium and coma.

Diagnosis

The history of diarrhea, the clinical picture and the serum electrolyte changes establish the presence of the syndrome. The cause is determined by a history of exposure, microscopic examination of the stool for the organism or leukocytes, cultures and febrile agglutinins. Barium enema and sigmoidoscopy and biopsy may be necessary in ulcerative colitis and amebiasis.

Treatment

Lactated potassic saline (Darrow's solution) (Table 7) is the replacement solution of choice, but a similar solution may be prepared using a liter of one half normal saline and adding 40 mEq. of potassium chloride and one ampule (44.6 mEq.) of sodium bicarbonate. Five percent dextrose in one half normal saline may be used as the basic solution to which the potassium and bicarbonate are added also. During the first four to six hours, 3 to 6 liters of this solution may be necessary depending on hourly monitoring of pH, blood volume and serum electrolytes.

Infants will require a different formula since their diarrhea fluid contains an average of 60 mEq./L. of sodium, 30 mEq./L. of potassium and 45 mEq./L. of chloride. Thus five percent dextrose in one-third normal saline with 20 mEq. of potassium chloride and one-half ampule (22.3 mEq.) of sodium bicarbonate added is a good formula for small infants (less than 12 Kg.). The fluid deficit is calculated on the basis of the known healthy weight (prior to illness) in Kilograms minus the admission weight. Large infants and children can be given 1,500 ml./sq. m. of body surface for maintenance, 2,400 ml./sq. m. of body surface for moderate fluid loss (10% weight loss) and 3,000 ml./sq. m. body surface for severe fluid loss (15% weight loss). See Table 8 (page 160) to calculate surface area.

Etiology

As mentioned above diarrhea may be secretory in cholera and *E. coli* infections, exudative in salmonella and shigella infections and a combination of both in ulcerative colitis and regional enteritis. Malabsorption syndrome (page 83), Zollinger-Ellison syndrome and carcinoid may also cause significant diarrhea to disturb electrolyte balance.

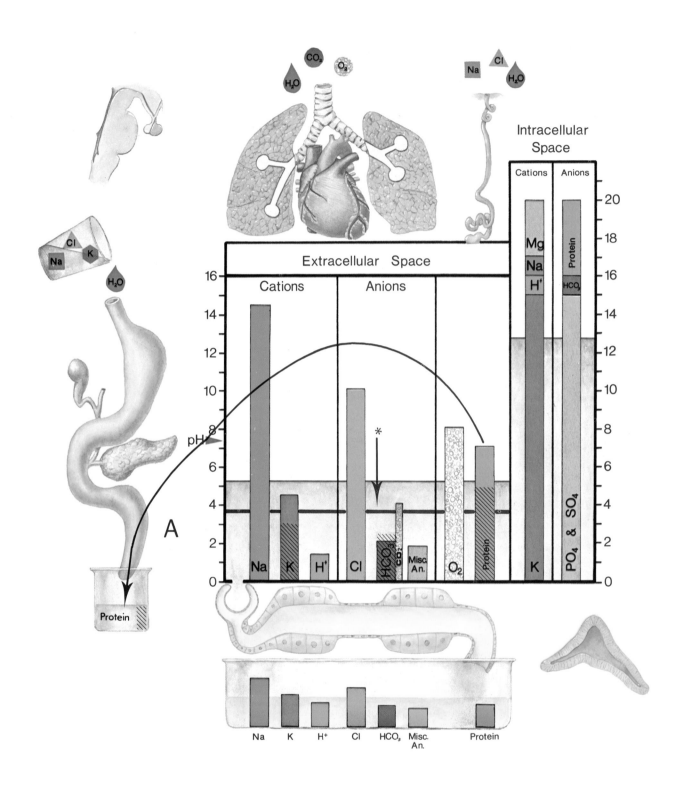

Summary of Abnormal Laboratory Findings

Serum Na—normal or
   increased
Serum K—decreased
Serum HCO_3^-—
   increased

Serum protein—
   decreased
Blood volume—
   decreased*

Protein-Losing Enteropathy

Pathophysiology

Under normal conditions 10 to 20 percent of the normal turnover of albumin may be associated with loss of protein through the gastrointestinal tract. In certain neoplastic (villous adenomas), degenerative and inflammatory conditions of the gastrointestinal tract 40 to 50 percent of all plasma proteins may be lost each day through the gastrointestinal tract (A). *Plasma protein decreases* with a concomitant *drop in circulatory* volume with escape of fluid extracellularly. Secondary aldosteronism as discussed under the nephrotic syndrome on page 93 may develop and lead to a low *serum potassium* with alkalosis and occasional hypernatremia. In villous adenomas, the mucous secretions contain a significant amount of potassium that aggravates the hypopotassemia.

Clinical Picture

The principal findings are bulk diarrhea and pitting edema. There may be generalized anasarca and severe weight loss. Other symptoms are of the underlying disorder.

Diagnosis

Serum protein electrophoresis shows a drop in serum albumin and all the globulin fractions. The most effective diagnostic method is the finding of excessive amounts of radioactive ^{131}I or ^{125}I labeled serum albumin in the stool following intravenous administration.

Treatment

This is usually directed toward the underlying disorder (steroids for ulcerative colitis, regional ileitis and Whipple's disease, etc.). Administration of salt-poor albumin is only temporarily effective. Mild diuretics may be given to partially correct the edema, but vigorous diuretic therapy should be resorted to only rarely. The hypokalemia should be corrected with an oral liquid potassium supplement.

Etiology

The list of disorders associated with this condition is long, but includes neoplasms such as carcinoma of the esophagus, stomach and colon; villous adenomas and lymphomas; inflammatory bowel disease; collagen disease; sprue; gastric atrophy and various cardiac disorders.

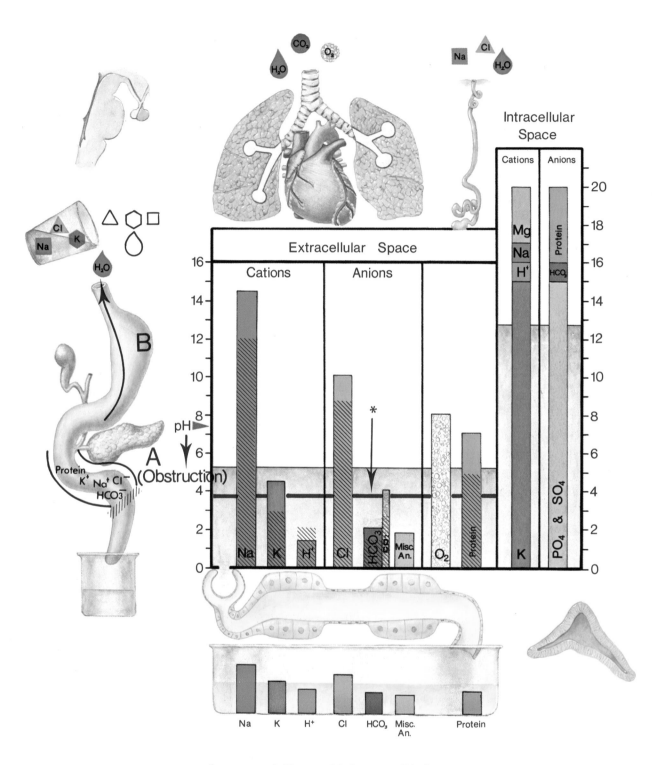

Summary of Abnormal Laboratory Findings

Serum Na—decreased

Serum K—decreased

Serum H+—increased

Serum Cl—decreased

Serum HCO3⁻—
    decreased

Serum protein—
    decreased

Blood volume—
    decreased*

Blood pH—decreased

Intestinal Obstruction

Pathophysiology

Upper intestinal obstruction associated with significant vomiting will produce a picture similar to that discussed under pyloric obstruction, page 99. With obstruction in the lower duodenum and beyond the ligament of Treitz, large amounts of fluid rich in sodium, potassium, chloride and bicarbonate will be lost into the intestinal lumen (A). Since more bicarbonate than chloride is lost there will be a metabolic acidosis. As much as three liters can be lost in this fashion during the first 24 hours in addition to losses resulting from vomiting (B). *Serum sodium, potassium, chloride* and *bicarbonate drop*. There is marked *hypovolemia*. The picture is similar to that seen in diarrhea. However, in intestinal obstruction large amounts of protein are lost through the inflamed bowel (A); thus, *serum protein drops* also.

Clinical Picture

There is colicky abdominal pain, nausea and vomiting, abdominal distention and constipation or obstipation. Dehydration and shock develop early. There is local or diffuse abdominal tenderness often with rebound tenderness signifying peritoneal irritation. Bowel sounds will be high pitched and active early, except in paralytic ileus, and diminished or absent later.

Diagnosis

This is established by a flat plate of the abdomen and the serum electrolyte changes. The hematocrit may be high unless there is associated blood loss. Lactic dehydrogenase is high in cases of mesenteric infarction. A bloody stool may signify intestinal infarction or intussusception.

Treatment

Most cases will require surgical intervention as soon as plasma volume is restored and shock controlled. In a few cases (adhesions, etc.) decompression with a Miller-Abbott tube will suffice until more adequate study of the problem can be undertaken. Lactated potassic saline (Darrow's solution) may be used to restore the intestinal losses along with one to two units of salt-free albumin or plasma to restore the protein. If there has been no hemorrhage the hematocrit may be used as a guide to the amount of fluid necessary with the following formula:

$$\text{Fluid deficit} = 0.6 \times \text{normal body weight in Kg.} - \left(\frac{\text{normal hematocrit}}{\text{measured hematocrit}} \times 0.6 \times \text{normal body wt. in Kg.} \right)$$

If there has been hemorrhage or the patient's hematocrit is assumed to be low prior to the development of the obstruction, blood volume determination will give some idea of the losses to be replaced immediately and frequent reevaluation may be necessary to keep pace. Continued losses through nasogastric suction or vomiting, insensible and sensible water loss and urine output must be replaced as well with appropriate solutions (page 157). Blood will have to be given in cases associated with hemorrhage. Calculation of water, sodium, potassium and bicarbonate losses with the formulas on page 156 is not often used, since their serum concentrations will not correlate well with the total body losses. However, if deficits of potassium and bicarbonate are significant they may be calculated and added to one-half normal saline as potassium chloride and sodium bicarbonate.

Etiology

A wide variety of vascular disease, neoplasms, malformations and inflammatory diseases may cause intestinal obstruction, but the most common are hernias and adhesions.

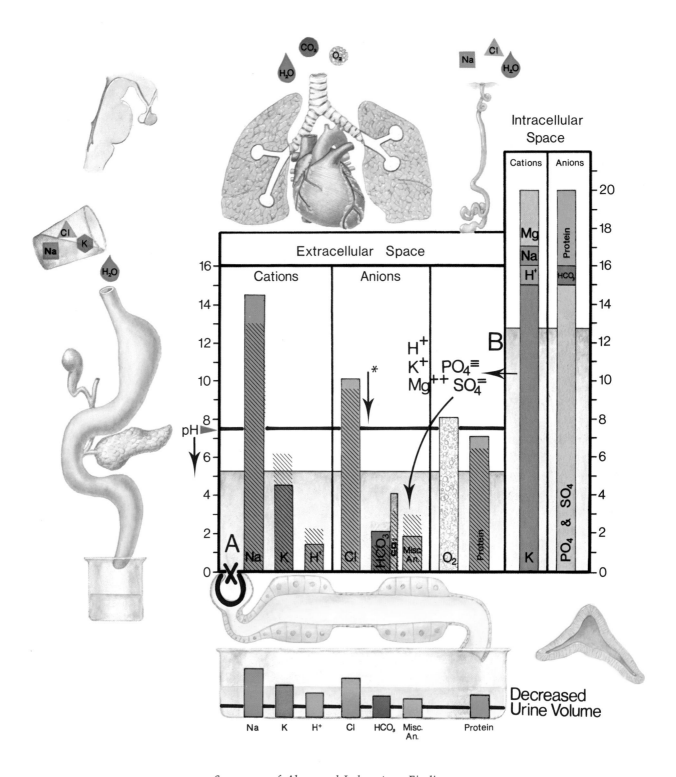

Summary of Abnormal Laboratory Findings

Serum Na—decreased
Serum K—increased
Serum H$^+$—increased
Serum Cl—decreased
Serum HCO$_3^-$—
   decreased

Serum miscellaneous
   anions—increased

Blood volume—
   increased*
Blood P$_{CO_2}$—decreased
Blood pH—decreased
Urine volume—
   decreased

Acute Renal Failure

Pathophysiology

In this disorder the excretion of water and all the major electrolytes of the body is blocked (A) and these accumulate in the body. However, the *serum potassium* is the only major electrolyte to *increase* in concentration. The *serum concentration of sodium and chloride decrease* because more water is retained than salt which results in a dilutional hyponatremia. *Blood and extracellular volume increase.* Because there is usually a reduction in food intake the body must rely on cell breakdown for energy. The cells release significant amounts of *hydrogen ion, potassium, magnesium, phosphates and sulfates* (B) and the level of all these rise in the serum because the kidney cannot excrete them. *Serum bicarbonate* is utilized to buffer these and other acid products of protein catabolism and because the diseased kidney cannot replace it, *its level drops.* This is usually not as severe as in other forms of metabolic acidosis. Although the lungs can compensate by hyperventilation and blow off more carbon dioxide, the *pH* nevertheless is usually *decreased.* Urine volume rarely exceeds 400 ml. a day. Cases of polyuric acute renal failure have been reported however.[15] The rise in serum phosphates (miscellaneous anions) may lower serum chloride, causing tetany.

Clinical Picture

In the early stages the symptoms are those of the underlying cause. Later there is edema, confusion and somnolence, nausea and vomiting, tremor and tetany and signs of congestive failure. Still later there may be convulsions and coma, arrhythmias (due to hyperkalemia) and pericarditis, uremic frost and sepsis.

Diagnosis

Oliguria is the most helpful clinical sign. This combined with the rise in serum potassium, urea, creatinine, phosphates and sulfates and a drop of pH and bicarbonate are usually diagnostic. The greatest difficulty is in differentiating between a prerenal and renal azotemia. A look at the urinary sediment for red cell and granular casts and other materials may help. The urine/plasma osmolality ratio is more helpful. In prerenal azotemia it is usually greater than 2:1 but in complete acute renal failure it is less than 1.1:1.[16] Varying degrees in between these limits usually mean partial renal failure. Urine sodium is usually above 40 mEq./L. in acute renal failure. Finally urine/plasma ratio of urea is more than 20:1 in prerenal azotemia and below that in acute renal failure.

A trial of mannitol or furosemide may be diagnostic as well as therapeutic (see below). Renal biopsy often will be necessary to determine the exact cause, but usually is done after the acute phase is past. If obstructive uropathy is suspected (and it usually should be until proved otherwise), cystoscopy and a retrograde pyelogram may be indicated.

Treatment

If the acute renal failure is thought to be due to prerenal causes (shock, dehydration, etc.) a trial of mannitol is worthwhile. One hundred milliliters of a 20 percent solution is given over a 10-minute period.[17] The urinary output should increase at least 50 percent in the next two hours; if not the dose may be repeated. Not more than 100 gm. of mannitol should be given in a 24-hour period. If the blood volume is good, furosemide up to a total dose of 1,000 mg. may be given, starting with 20 to 40 mg. I.V. and increasing until a good response is accomplished. If these measures have been unsuccessful or if it has been determined at the outset that severe tubular necrosis is present, conservative therapy may be undertaken as follows:

1. **Fluid Requirements.** Replace insensible water loss — gains from metabolism + urine output + vomiting or other losses. This is usually 400 to 600 ml. a day. Daily weight is checked to be sure there is no gain.

2. **Caloric Requirements.** Give 100 to 150 gm. of carbohydrate daily either orally as equal parts of Karo and ginger ale with lemon flavor or intravenously by continuous slow infusion of 50 percent dextrose and water into the vena cava.

3. **Hyperkalemia.** This may be controlled in the acute situation by intravenous 50 percent dextrose and insulin (to drive potassium back into the cell) or calcium gluconate administration. It may be prevented by proper attention to caloric requirements and Kayexalate (ion-exchange resins) orally or by enemas. If these measures fail peritoneal or renal dialysis must be resorted to (hyperkalemia is the prime indication for dialysis).

4. **Metabolic Acidosis.** This need not be treated unless the serum bicarbonate drops below 15 mEq./L. Then only small doses of sodium bicarbonate are given with careful monitoring of the blood gases. This may bring down the serum potassium as well.

5. **Water Intoxication.** A phlebotomy may be performed if there is associated congestive heart failure. Otherwise hypertonic saline (3-5%) is given in acute cases. Water restriction is the best treatment for

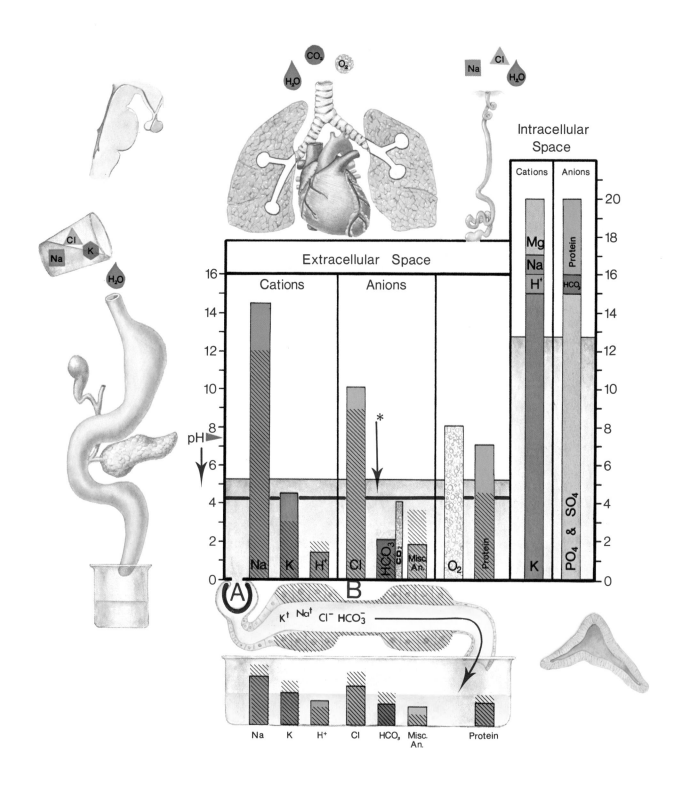

Summary of Abnormal Laboratory Findings

Serum Na—decreased
   or normal
Serum H⁺—increased
Serum K—normal,
   increased or
   decreased

Serum Cl—decreased or
   normal
Serum HCO₃⁻—
   decreased
Serum protein—
   decreased

Serum miscellaneous
   anions—increased
Blood pH—decreased
Blood volume—
   decreased*

moderate cases. Dialysis may have to be resorted to when other measures fail.

6. Hypocalcemia. This is prevented by oral administration of aluminum hydroxide gel to inhibit the reabsorption of phosphates. If tetany develops, calcium gluconate is given intravenously.

Active treatment is in the form of peritoneal and renal dialysis, for which a nephrologist should be consulted. Steroids, antibiotics and other measures are resorted to in treating the underlying cause. Digitalis is used in secondary pulmonary edema.

In the *diuretic phase* urine output and electrolytes are measured every four hours and the intravenous fluid prescription altered appropriately.

Etiology

Acute renal failure may result from a variety of drugs, poisons, heavy metals, transfusions or other hemolytic reactions, shock, dehydration, glomerulonephritis, or obstructive uropathy.

Chronic Renal Failure

Pathophysiology

The rise in blood urea, creatinine and uric acid can best be explained by the reduced glomerular filtration rate (A), whereas the electrolyte derangement of chronic renal insufficiency can best be explained by a loss of the kidney's regulatory powers in water, electrolyte and acid-base equilibrium. This will not be lost until 70 to 80 percent of the nephron population has been destroyed. Thus serum electrolytes may be normal in most cases of chronic renal disease.

In cases with significant tubular damage (B) the kidney loses its ability to reabsorb water and electrolytes selectively and to produce bicarbonate in controlling acid-base equilibrium. The tubules fail to respond to the salt-retaining stimulus of aldosterone or the water-retaining stimulus of ADH. Thus *serum sodium may drop* and *blood volume may decrease,* especially when there is dietary restriction. On the other hand major increments of dietary water, sodium, chloride and potassium may not be tolerated because of the reduced glomerular filtration rate and their serum levels may rise. Replacement of plasma bicarbonate and excretion of hydrogen ion may cease, with consequent metabolic acidosis. This along with the impaired excretion of inorganic acids such as *sulfates* and *phosphates* (miscellaneous anions) causes a *rise in serum hydrogen ions* and a *drop in serum bicarbonate.* Tubular reabsorption of potassium may be impaired and *serum potassium may drop* on dietary restriction or when there is vomiting or diarrhea.

Clinical Picture

Chronic anorexia, weakness, weight loss and occasional nausea and vomiting are the usual symptoms. In more severe cases there is somnolence, convulsions, peripheral neuropathy, skin pigmentation and pruritis, purpura and hemorrhages, congestive heart failure and anemia.

Diagnosis

The finding of increased BUN, creatinine and uric acid with the above electrolyte alterations is usually diagnostic. The differentiation from prerenal azotemia has already been discussed under acute renal failure, page 107. Cystoscopy and retrograde pyelography may be necessary to exclude obstruction uropathy. Other diagnostic procedures, such as urine cultures, antinuclear antibody test, and renal biopsy should be directed at establishing an etiologic diagnosis.

Treatment

Before considering renal dialysis or transplant, certain conservative measures may control the average patient for some time.

Diet. With BUN values above 200 mg. a nonprotein diet should be given. When the BUN is between 100 and 200 mg. a 30-gm. protein diet can be prescribed. The fluid intake is increased by 500 ml. increments daily until a similar increase in urine output does not occur. Then the intake is kept at the level of the previous day. A urine output of 2 to 2.5 L. is usually optimal as long as edema and weight gain do not occur. The grams of protein permissible in the diet may be calculated by ordering a 24-hour urine urea and multiplying the value by three.

Hyperpotassemia, hypocalcemia and hyperphosphatemia are treated as described on page 107 in acute renal failure.

Chronic metabolic acidosis is treated by administering sodium bicarbonate or sodium citrate tablets daily.

Anemia is treated with packed cells only if the hemoglobin drops below 7 gm. or if there is shock or hemorrhage.

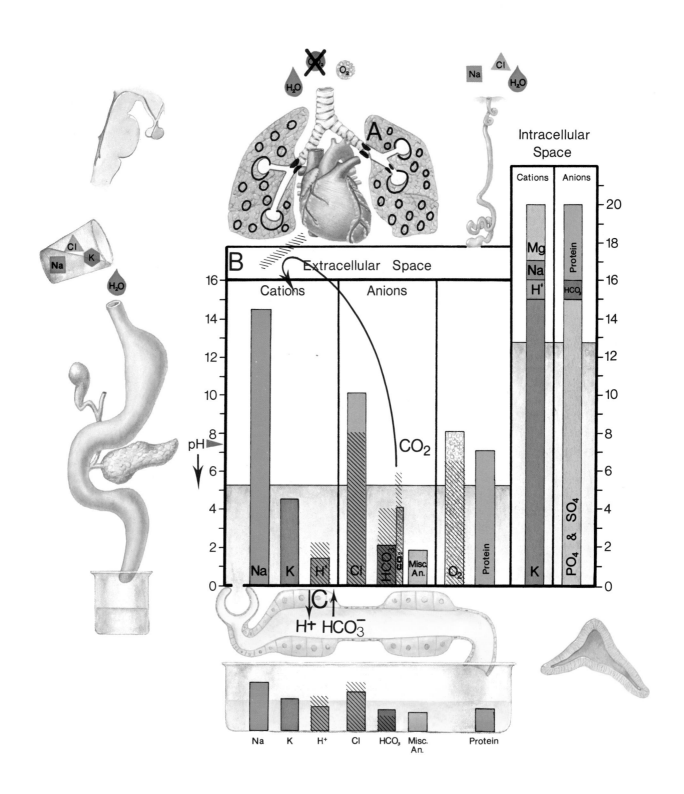

Summary of Abnormal Laboratory Findings

Serum H⁺—increased	or increased*
Serum Cl—decreased	Blood P_{CO_2}—increased
Serum HCO₃⁻—	Blood P_{O_2}—decreased
increased	or normal
Blood volume—normal	Blood pH—decreased

Congestive heart failure is treated with low doses of digitalis because its renal excretion is impaired. Edema may be treated with furosemide or ethacrynic acid.

Salt depletion may be treated with salt tablets. Other treatment (antibiotics, steroids) is directed at the specific cause.

Etiology

Common causes of chronic renal failure are pyelonephritis, glomerulonephritis, nephrosclerosis, polycystic kidneys, collagen diseases, and obstructive uropathy. More detailed lists may be found in standard textbooks.

Pulmonary Emphysema

Pathophysiology

Obstruction of the bronchi and bronchioles (A) leads to alveolar hypoventilation, bullae and poor capillary perfusion of some alveoli that are ventilated adequately. *Carbon dioxide "excretion"* is impaired (B) and so its level *rises* in the blood. This leads to a *rise in hydrogen ion* because of the formation of carbonic acid by the following reaction:

$$CO_2 + H_2O \longrightarrow H^+ + HCO_3^-$$

Thus *pH drops*. The kidney acts to compensate for the respiratory acidosis by excreting hydrogen ion and retaining bicarbonate through the carbonic anhydrase system (C). Serum *chloride drops* since it is excreted with the hydrogen ions and ammonia by the following reaction:

$$NH_3 + H^+ + Cl^- \longrightarrow NH_4Cl$$

Accordingly the urine is usually acid. In later stages and in acute exacerbations *arterial* P_{O_2} *drops* because of severe ventilatory insufficiency and pulmonary fibrosis.

Clinical Picture

In the chronic stages there may be only mild cough and hyperventilation, slight cyanosis, clubbing and moderate weight loss. In the acute stages there may be somnolence and coma, productive cough, severe cyanosis, edema, and other signs of right heart failure. Chest examination reveals hyperresonance throughout the lung, increased A-P diameter, diminished alveolar breathing, increased bronchial breathing and sibilant and sonorous rales on expiration.

Diagnosis

Arterial blood gases, serum electrolytes, chest films and pulmonary function studies will establish the diagnosis.

Treatment

In the chronic stages, bronchodilators, such as aminophylline and ephedrine, expectorants (saturated solution of potassium iodide, etc.) and antibiotics (tetracyclines, etc.) are useful. Home IPPB (intermittent positive pressure breathing) with saline, isoproterenol (Isuprel) and acetylcysteine (Mucomyst) in various combinations may be necessary. During the acute stages semicontinuous or continuous IPPB with saline, isoproterenol and acetylcysteine through an endotracheal tube or tracheostomy may be necessary. Oxygen therapy should be as low as possible but enough to keep the blood P_{O_2} above 60 mm. Hg. Sodium bicarbonate is rarely necessary unless pH is very low and tromethamine (tris[hydroxymethyl]aminomethane) would be safer.[18] Hourly determinations of blood gases and serum electrolytes may be necessary to spot post-hypercapnic metabolic alkalosis early. This can be treated with potassium chloride or hypertonic saline. Digitalis and diuretics may be necessary if significant right heart failure develops, but these patients respond poorly to digitalis. Phlebotomy may be necessary if there is severe polycythemia.

Etiology

Pulmonary emphysema may occur in pneumoconiosis, silicosis and bronchial asthma, although most cases are idiopathic. Respiratory acidosis may occur in pneumonia, pneumothorax, poliomyelitis, barbiturate intoxication and during anesthesia. It also occurs in the end stages of shock.

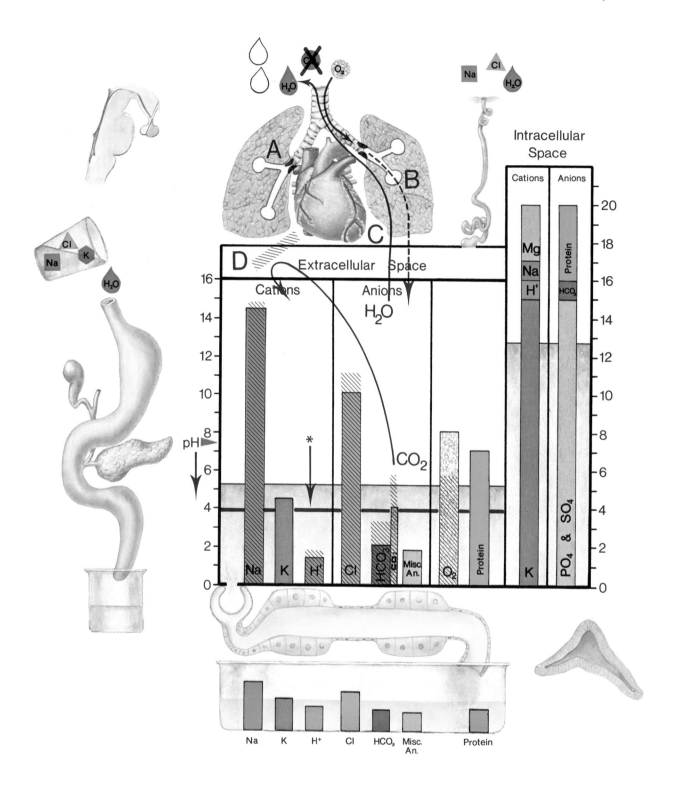

Summary of Abnormal Laboratory Findings

Serum Na—increased
Serum H⁺—increased
Serum Cl—increased
Serum HCO₃⁻—
    decreased early,
    increased late

Blood volume—
    decreased*
Blood P$_{O_2}$—decreased

Blood P$_{CO_2}$—decreased
    early, increased late
Blood pH—increased
    early, decreased late.

Asthmatic Attack

Pathophysiology

Bronchospasm and thick tenacious mucus obstruct the respiratory passages (A) in this disorder and lead to dyspnea and hyperventilation. In the very early stages the compensatory mechanisms may be adequate so that blood oxygen content may be normal while P_{CO_2} *falls*, carbonic acid decreases and *hydrogen ion drops with a reciprocal rise in pH*. After the attack continues for a few hours there is more severe airway obstruction and an alteration in the perfusion/ventilation ratio. Thus *blood oxygen drops* since oxygen cannot get to the blood (B). With prolonged hyperventilation large amounts of water are lost via the lungs (C). Thus *circulatory volume drops* and serum *sodium* and *chloride rise*. As the attack continues, further obstruction of the bronchi and bronchioles becomes so severe that carbon dioxide excretion is impaired (D) and this rises in the blood. Compensatory mechanisms such as retention of bicarbonate occur so that the electrolyte picture is identical to that in pulmonary emphysema on page 111.

Clinical Picture

Hyperventilation, audible wheezing, cyanosis and cough productive of thick mucoid sputum are the usual findings. Examination of the chest reveals generalized wheezing, rhonchi, prolonged expiration and hyperventilation. Signs of right heart failure may develop late. Pale bluish mucoid turbinates may be noted on examination of the nasal passages.

Diagnosis

Previous history of asthma, hay fever or allergies coupled with nasal or sputum smears for eosinophils may be all that is necessary to differentiate bronchial asthma from other forms of pulmonary emphysema. The blood gases and electrolytes in this early stage of an attack may be confused with those of pulmonary embolism, pneumonia, shock or the hyperventilation syndrome, but these can usually be differentiated by lung scans, chest roentgenograms, blood pressure and psychiatric history respectively. Skin tests to determine the specific allergen should be undertaken later.

Treatment

Early attacks are treated with epinephrine (0.3-0.5 mg.) intravenously or subcutaneously and may be given as often as every 20 minutes for three to five doses. Oxygen therapy by ventimask at 28 percent and intravenous 5 percent dextrose and water are begun simultaneously to combat anoxia and dehydration (from the increased amounts of insensible water loss via the lungs). If epinephrine is unsuccessful, aminophylline is given 4 to 6 mg./Kg. intravenously at 20 mg./min. When both these measures fail (and sometimes simultaneously) corticosteroids in the form of dexamethasone 10 to 15 mg. intravenously every two to four hours should be given. It may be necessary to continue this for 24 to 28 hours and gradually taper the dose for three to four more days. Some physicians start antibiotics at the same time they begin corticosteroids in case there is an infectious component to the asthma. Other therapeutic methods such as IPPB, sedatives and antihistamines may be necessary. Endotracheal entubation or tracheotomy should not be delayed when drug therapy is only minimally successful or when the situation seems urgent. Sodium bicarbonate is rarely required to combat the respiratory acidosis and even then should be used sparingly.

Etiology

Pollens of ragweed, grass, trees and other plants are the principal offenders, but almost any substance light enough to become airborne and small enough to be inhaled can cause asthma.

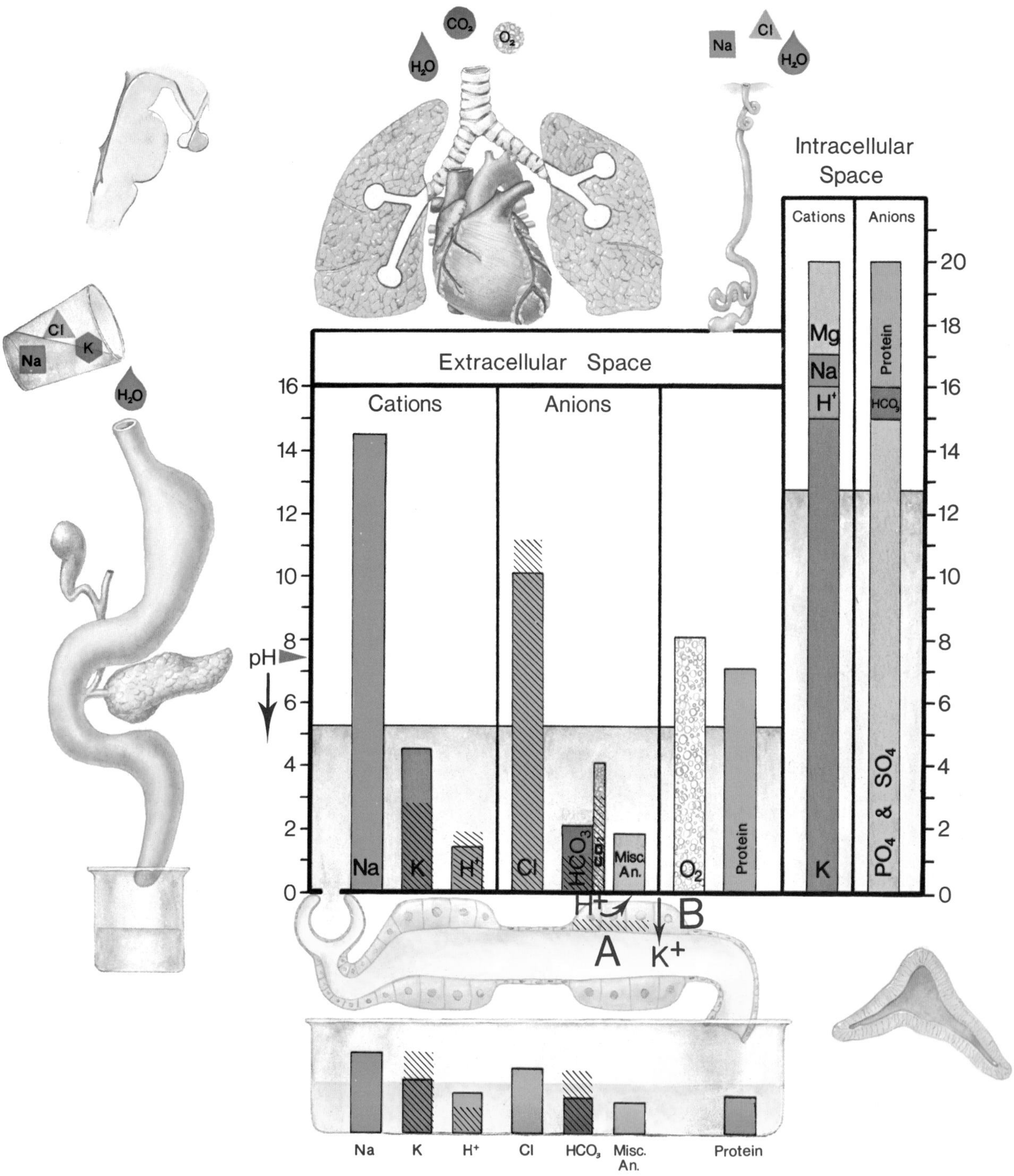

Summary of Abnormal Laboratory Findings

Serum Na—normal or decreased

Serum K—decreased

Serum H⁺—increased

Serum Cl—increased

Serum HCO_3^-—decreased

Blood pH—decreased

Urine pH—increased

Classical Renal Tubular Acidosis

Pathophysiology

In this hereditary disorder there is a distal tubular defect (A) in the secretion of hydrogen ions in exchange for tubular sodium.[19] Thus *hydrogen ion rises* and *pH drops* in the blood while less sodium is reabsorbed as bicarbonate and serum *bicarbonate falls*. The tubules, unable to secrete hydrogen ion for sodium, secrete more potassium in exchange for sodium instead (B). Consequently the *serum potassium drops. Serum chloride rises* to make up the deficit in anions caused by the low bicarbonate. Unlike chronic renal failure, glomerular filtration rate is not usually reduced significantly so that the excretion of sulfates, phosphates and other acids is unimpaired. Thus *serum miscellaneous anions* are not increased. The acidosis induces hypercalciuria and hypocalcemia as well.

Clinical Picture

The chronic acidosis may cause anorexia, lethargy and hyperventilation. The hypopotassemia may induce weakness, muscular paralysis and cardiac arrhythmias. There may be osteomalacia growth retardation and nephrolithiasis (from the hypercalciuria). These patients are also susceptible to pyelonephritis.

Diagnosis

The serum electrolytes, pH, and a persistently alkaline urine without azotemia (in most cases) are important diagnostic features. Differentiation from bicarbonate wastage renal tubular acidosis (page 117) can be made by observing that the classical form improves quickly on the administration of sodium bicarbonate. The urine pH is also invariably high in the classical form.

Treatment

From 50 to 100 ml. of Shohl's solution (140 gm. citric acid and 98 gm. of hydrated crystalline salt of sodium citrate in 1,000 ml. of water) is given daily by mouth in three divided doses. A potassium supplement is also given. Supplemental calcium or vitamin D is not required. During a fulminant crisis, infusions of sodium bicarbonate and potassium chloride may be necessary.

Etiology

This disorder is probably inherited as a mendelian dominant trait. It may also occur in dysproteinemic states.

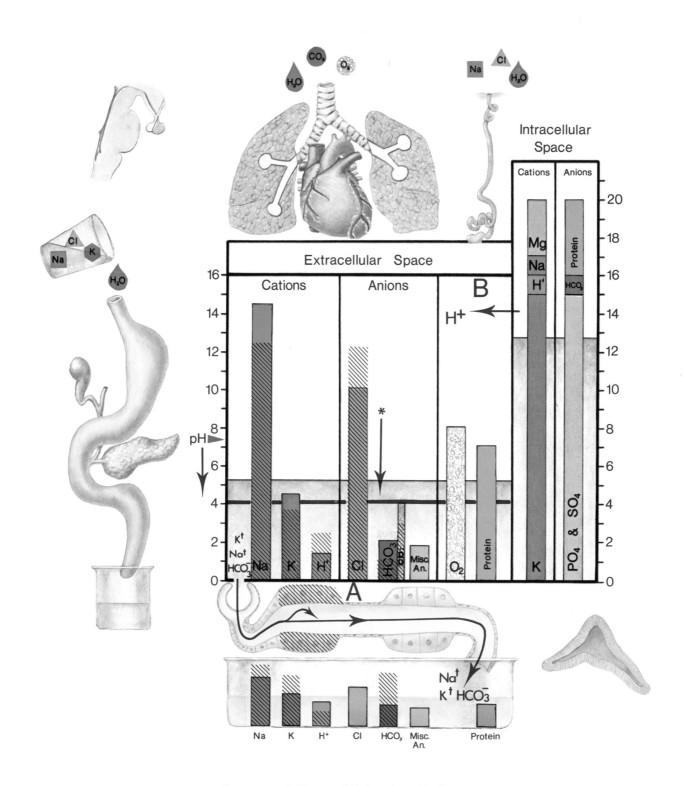

Summary of Abnormal Laboratory Findings

Serum Na—decreased   Blood volume—
Serum K—decreased   decreased*
Serum H$^+$—increased   Blood pH—decreased
Serum Cl—increased   Urine pH—increased
Serum HCO$_3^-$—   Urine HCO$_3^-$—
    decreased   markedly increased

Bicarbonate Wastage Renal Tubular Acidosis

Pathophysiology

In this disorder the proximal tubule (A) is unable to reabsorb bicarbonate. *Serum bicarbonate drops.* Both *potassium* and *sodium* are excreted with the bicarbonate in the urine and their *plasma levels drop.* *Blood volume drops* due to the tremendous loss of sodium. *Hydrogen ions* move out of the cells (B) to make up the deficit in cations and thus their plasma level *rises. Serum chloride rises* to make up the deficit in chloride ions. As in the classic form there may be hypercalciuria and hypocalcemia. Unlike chronic renal failure, phosphate and sulfate excretion is unimpaired and so *serum miscellaneous anions do not rise.*

Clinical Picture

This is similar to the "classic form" (page 115) unless it is part of the Fanconi syndrome in which case the features of that syndrome will also be present.[14]

Diagnosis

The serum electrolytes, low serum pH and high pH of the urine help establish the diagnosis. In addition there may be aminoaciduria and glucosuria. To differentiate this type from the classical form, the serum electrolytes and pH are observed after sodium bicarbonate administration. In the bicarbonate wastage form the serum electrolytes and pH fail to change significantly after sodium bicarbonate.

Treatment

This is similar to treatment of the classical form except that large doses of vitamin D and calcium phosphate are given as well.

Etiology

This condition may be primary or secondary to a Fanconi syndrome, heavy metal poisoning, dysproteinemia or hereditary fructose intolerance.[19]

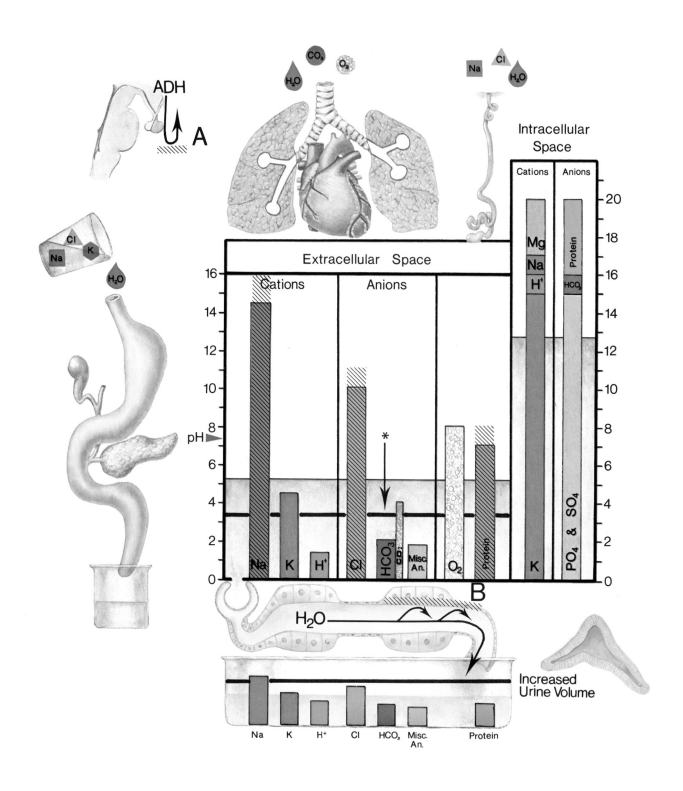

Summary of Abnormal Laboratory Findings

Serum Na—increased   Blood volume—
Serum Cl—increased   decreased*
Serum protein—   Urine volume—
    increased   markedly increased

Diabetes Insipidus

Pathophysiology

In this disorder there is failure of the supraoptic nucleus and neurohypophyseal system to produce or release ADH (A). Without ADH the distal and collecting tubules fail to reabsorb water (B). *Blood volume decreases* while *urine volume increases* (sometimes to 15 liters a day.) The reduced blood volume stimulates aldosterone production and sodium is retained. Both serum *sodium* and *chloride* rise. Thirst and polydipsia fail to remedy the situation.

Clinical Picture

There is dehydration, thirst, polydipsia, polyuria and nocturia of abrupt onset. The patient characteristically desires cold water.

Diagnosis

Continued polyuria with water restriction and the intravenous infusion of hypertonic saline (Hickey-Hare test) are helpful, but the cessation of polyuria with vasopressin administration is probably the best test and helps rule out nephrogenic diabetes insipidus. Roentgenograms of the skull and other tests may disclose the etiology. The ratio of urine to plasma osmolality will be 1:1 or less.

Treatment

Administration of 0.5 ml. of nasopressin (Pitressin tannate, 5 units/ml.) every two days will control most cases. During acute stages aqueous Pitressin (20 units/ml.) may be given subcutaneously.

Etiology

The idiopathic type accounts for 50 percent of cases. The rest may be due to pituitary tumors, basal skull fractures, granulomas, cerebrovascular disease, encephalitis and intracranial surgery.

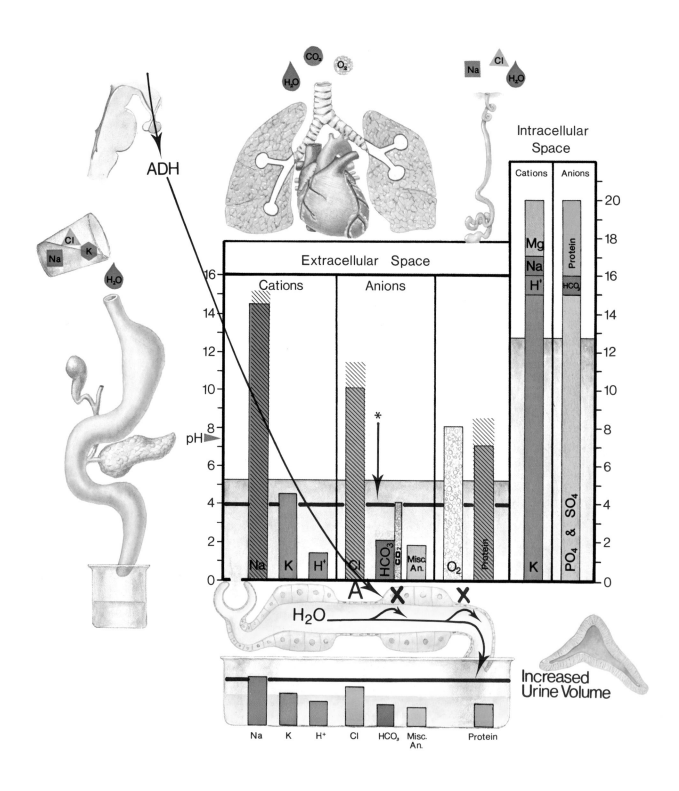

Summary of Abnormal Laboratory Findings

Serum Na—increased   Blood volume—
Serum Cl—increased   decreased*
Serum protein—   Urine volume—
    increased   moderately to
                                markedly increased

Nephrogenic Diabetes Insipidus

Pathophysiology

In this hereditary disorder there is adequate production and release of ADH, but the distal and collecting tubules fail to respond to it (A). Thus water is not reabsorbed (just as in diabetes insipidus) and urine volume rises while *blood volume drops*. Serum *sodium* and *chloride* rise so that the electrolyte picture is identical to "neurohypophyseal" diabetes insipidus.

Clinical Picture

There is moderate dehydration, thirst, polydipsia, polyuria and nocturia. There is a high incidence of mental retardation.

Diagnosis

Failure of the diuresis to respond to intravenous Pitressin differentiates this condition from "neuro- hypophyseal" diabetes insipidus. Renal biopsy is not helpful in the hereditary form.

Treatment

An isocaloric diluted whole milk formula seems best for optimal growth and to reduce the time spent drinking.[20] Thiazide diuretics are also useful.

Etiology

Besides the hereditary type, acquired nephrogenic diabetes insipidus may result from lithium carbonate, demeclocycline and methoxyflurane anesthesia. Hypercalcemia and hypokalemia may cause a partial nephrogenic diabetes insipidus. Chronic glomerulonephritis and other causes of chronic renal failure (page 109) are associated with renal tubular unresponsiveness to ADH.

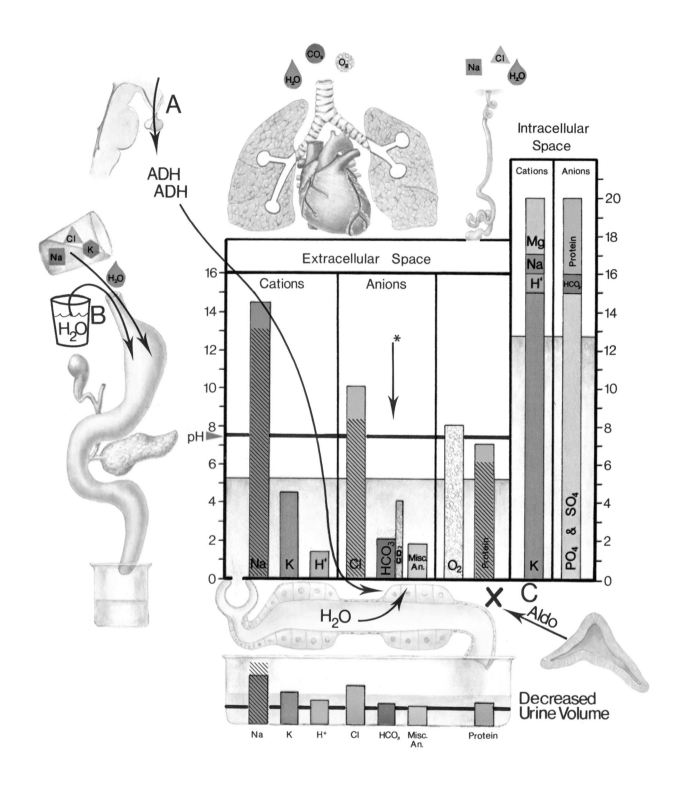

Summary of Abnormal Laboratory Findings

Serum Na—decreased   Blood volume—
Serum Cl—decreased   increased*
Serum protein—   Urine volume—
    decreased   decreased or normal
                             Urine Na—increased

Inappropriate ADH Secretion

Pathophysiology

In this group of disorders, secretion of antidiuretic hormone (A) and consequent renal conservation of water is not associated with a significant reduction in water ingestion (B). Thus *plasma, extracellular, and intracellular volume expand. Serum sodium* and *chloride decrease* from the dilutional effect and also from a reduction of aldosterone secretion (C) brought about by the effect of the increased plasma volume on the renin-angiotensin system. The expanded plasma and extracellular volume also inhibits the proximal tubular reabsorption of sodium.[2]

Clinical Picture

There are signs of water intoxication including delirium, coma and seizures. Although the volume of fluid is increased throughout the body, frank edema may not be present. Other symptoms are of the underlying disorder.

Diagnosis

In most cases urine osmolality will be significantly higher than plasma osmolality (>1:1 ratio). However some cases may show an isotonic or hypotonic urine. Urinary sodium excretion is usually 25 mEq./24 hr. or more on a normal intake.

Treatment

Water restriction is the best treatment. In acute cases in which water intoxication is extreme, an infusion of hypertonic saline (3-5%), urea, or mannitol may be necessary. The urea and mannitol may induce a solute diuresis.

Etiology

Most cases are associated with bronchogenic carcinomas, tuberculosis, and cerebral lesions such as skull fractures, subdural hematomas, brain tumors, cerebrovascular disease of all kinds and postoperative conditions.[2]

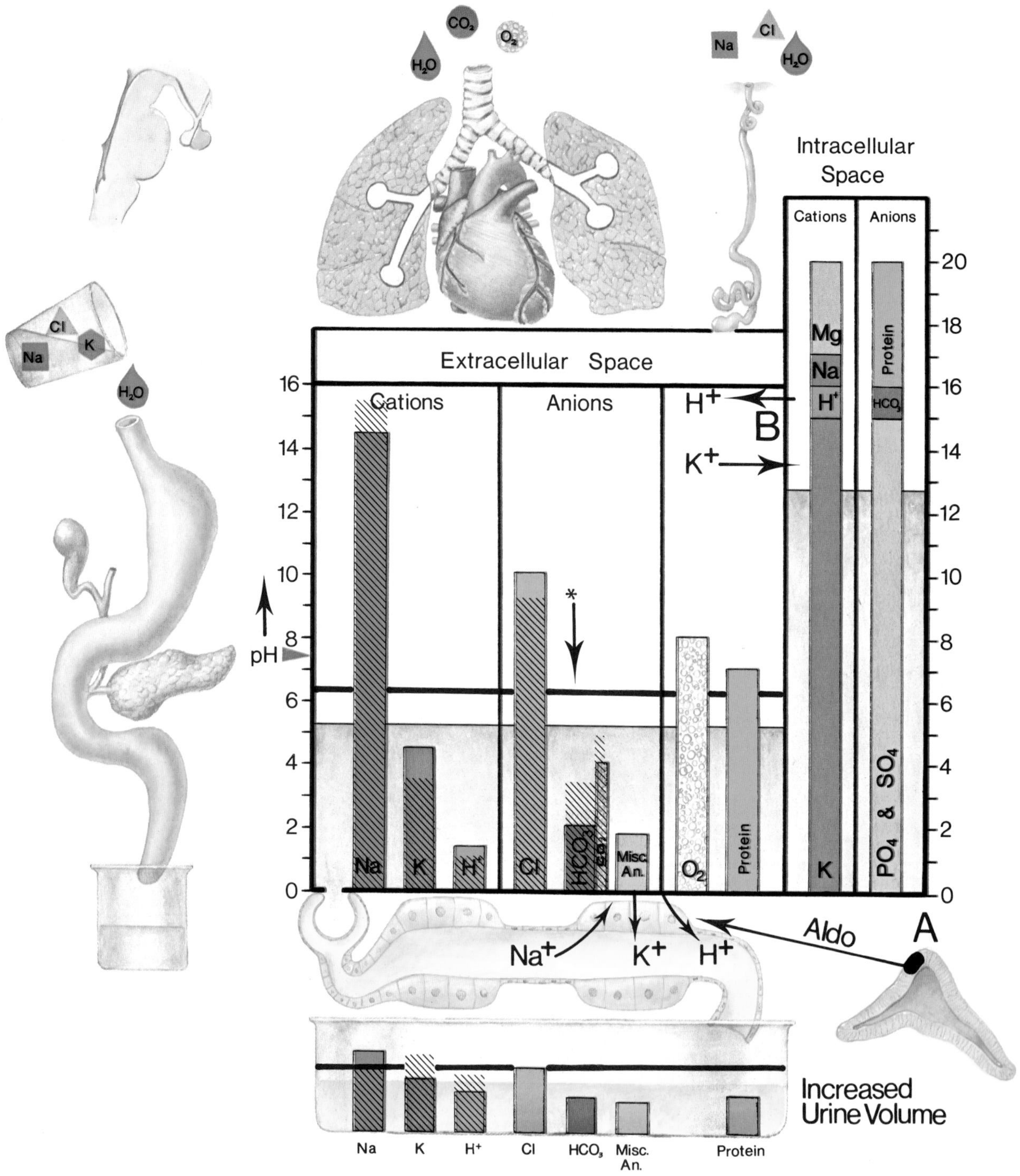

Summary of Abnormal Laboratory Findings

Serum Na—increased
Serum K—decreased
Serum H⁺—decreased
Serum HCO₃⁻—
  increased
Serum Cl—decreased

Blood volume—
  increased*
Urine Na—decreased
Urine K—increased
Urine volume—
  increased

Primary Aldosteronism

Pathophysiology

Secretion of excessive aldosterone by the adrenal cortex (A) activates the distal tubule to reabsorb large amounts of sodium in exchange for potassium and hydrogen ions. As a result *serum sodium* and bicarbonate *increase* while *serum hydrogen ions* and *potassium drop*. The resulting metabolic alkalosis with a *rise in pH* forces potassium into the cell in exchange for hydrogen ion (B) further aggravating the hypopotassemia. The resulting hypernatremia may stimulate the supraoptic nucleus to release ADH and *increase blood volume*, but its action on the distal and collecting tubules is antagonized by aldosterone so that polyuria may develop despite these events.

Clinical Picture

Although the patient may complain of weakness, fatigue, tetany, and polyuria, the usual finding is moderate hypertension. In many patients symptoms are absent or mild.

Diagnosis

In the routine hypertensive workup, three daily serum potassiums are done (with diuretic therapy discontinued). If these are low or low normal then a 24-hour urine potassium with the patient on a normal diet is done. If this is in excess of 20 to 30 mEq. a day primary aldosteronism is likely. Then a detailed study of the plasma renin is undertaken. After restoring electrolyte balance with a 100 mEq. potassium and 10 mEq. sodium diet, plasma renins are done in the supine and upright positions and 24-hour urinary aldosterone excretion rates are measured. On two consecutive days thereafter the patient is given 2 liters of isotonic saline over a four-hour period. The aldosterone secretory rate and plasma renin are measured the morning after the second day. Plasma renin will remain low but aldosterone will remain high or increase after this test. This procedure will vary from laboratory to laboratory so that the endocrinologist or pathologist in charge should be consulted. Adrenal venography has been most successful in outlining this type of adrenal tumor.[21]

Treatment

Surgical removal of the involved gland (or both glands in case of hyperplasia) is the treatment of choice. Until this can be accomplished, a low-salt, high potassium diet and spironolactone (150-200 mg./day) are given.

Etiology

Most cases are due to an adenoma, hyperplasia or carcinoma (rare) as in other adrenal tumors.

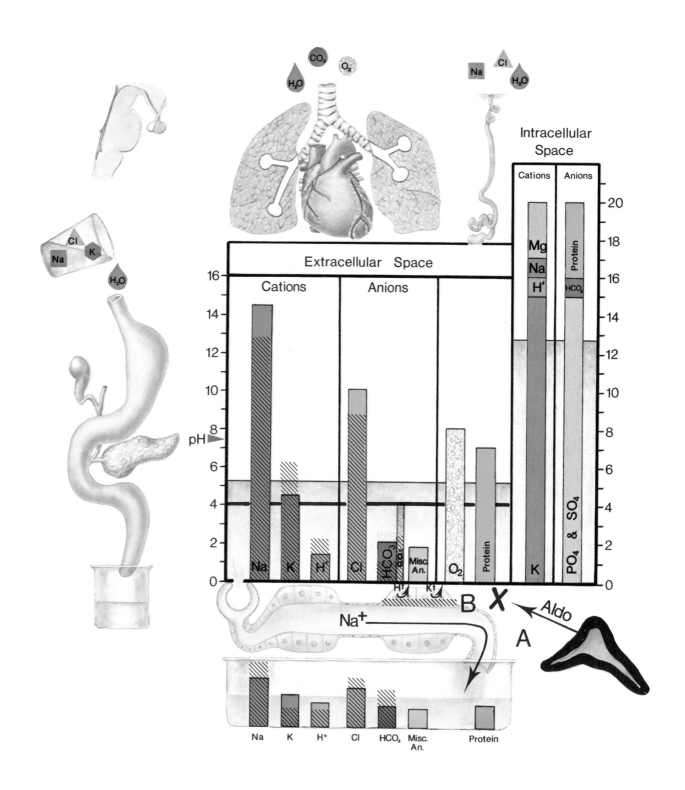

Summary of Abnormal Laboratory Findings

Serum Na—decreased	Blood volume— decreased*	Urine Na—increased or normal
Serum K—increased		
Serum Cl—decreased	Urine volume—normal or decreased	Urine K—decreased
Serum HCO$_3^-$—normal or decreased		Urine Cl—increased

Adrenal Cortical Insufficiency

Pathophysiology

In this disorder there is insufficient aldosterone (and possibly other mineralocorticoid) secretion (A) to induce the distal tubule to reabsorb sodium in exchange for potassium and hydrogen ions (B). Thus *serum sodium drops* while *serum potassium* and *hydrogen ion rise.* Large amounts of sodium chloride and some bicarbonate are lost in the urine. The salt takes with it substantial quantities of water and so *blood volume drops.* However, the lack of aldosterone inhibition of ADH prevents severe dehydration.

Clinical Picture

There is weakness, anorexia, weight loss, nausea and vomiting, hypotension and occasional attacks of hypoglycemia. Diffuse hyperpigmentation plus bluish-black patches on the mucous membranes are characteristic.

Diagnosis

The Robinson-Power-Kepler test is still a useful screening procedure. Following a period of fluid restriction, a water load is administered (20 ml./Kg.), and hourly urine volumes are recorded. Less than 1,000 ml. urine output in the four hours following the water load suggests adrenal cortical insufficiency. Plasma cortisol levels before and after ACTH are more specific. These of course are low and remain after ACTH.

Treatment

Most patients are controlled on 30 to 40 mg. of hydrocortisone daily. If the electrolytes are not brought back to normal, a mineralocorticoid such as 9-alpha-fluorohydrocortisone is given (0.1 to 0.2 mg. daily).

Etiology

Idiopathic atrophy accounts for the majority of cases seen, but granulomatous disease such as tuberculosis and histoplasmosis may be the cause in some cases.

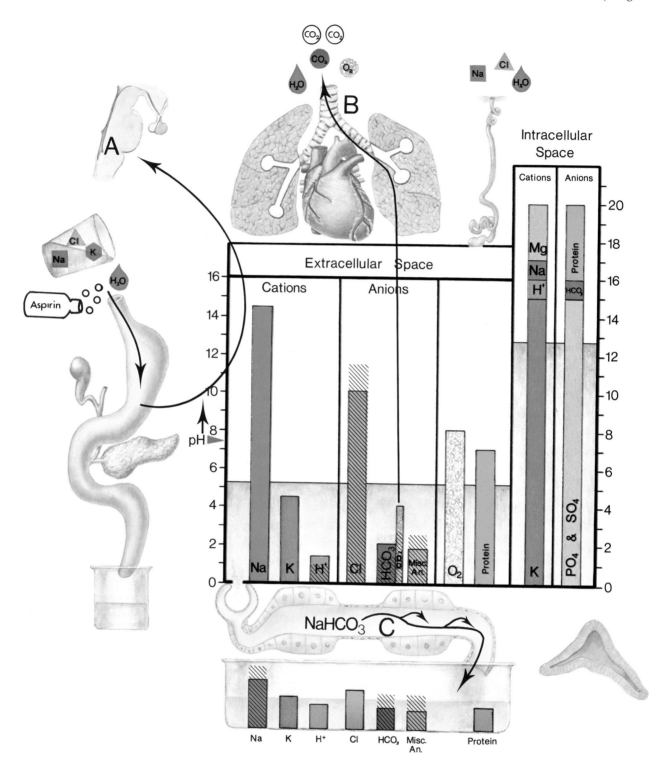

Summary of Abnormal Laboratory Findings

Serum Na—normal or
    decreased
Serum K—normal or
    decreased
Serum H⁺—decreased
    early, increased late

Serum Cl—increased
Serum HCO₃⁻—
    decreased
Blood Pco₂—decreased

Blood pH—increased
    early, decreased late
Urine Na—increased
Urine HCO₃⁻—
    increased

Salicylate Toxicity

Pathophysiology

Large doses of salicylates stimulate the respiratory center (A) causing hyperventilation. There is increased excretion of carbon dioxide via the lungs (B) and its *blood level drops*. Thus blood carbonic acid and hydrogen ions also *decrease* while *pH rises*. To compensate for the loss of hydrogen ions and carbon dioxide the kidney reabsorbs less *bicarbonate* (C) and its *blood level drops also*. The *serum chloride increases* to make up the deficit in anions. With large doses of salicylates *serum miscellaneous anions* may *increase* either directly (due to the salicylic acid) or indirectly from ketones formed when the salicylates block carbohydrate metabolism. Thus a metabolic acidosis may develop later.

Clinical Picture

Hyperventilation, nausea and vomiting, diaphoresis, confusion and coma are seen. Tetany may develop.

Diagnosis

The electrolyte picture is suggestive but not diagnostic, and blood and urine salicylate levels must be determined. Most symptomatic patients will have blood levels over 35 mg. per 100 ml.

Treatment

Lavage with sodium bicarbonate is performed and activated charcoal is administered to reduce salicylate absorption. Isotonic saline is administered to correct the alkalosis and diurese the salicylates. Mannitol (10-15% Osmitrol) may be given to remove the salicylates concomitantly (via another I.V. catheter) or once the alkalosis is brought under control. A rebreathing bag or mixtures of oxygen and carbon dioxide by nose are given to help correct the alkalosis. Blood gases are tested frequently to detect early metabolic acidosis; then the bicarbonate deficit is calculated and half of this is given before a reevaluation of blood gases and electrolytes is done. Peritoneal and renal dialysis may be necessary in some cases.

Etiology

The hyperventilation syndrome, fever, high altitude and head trauma may produce the same picture.

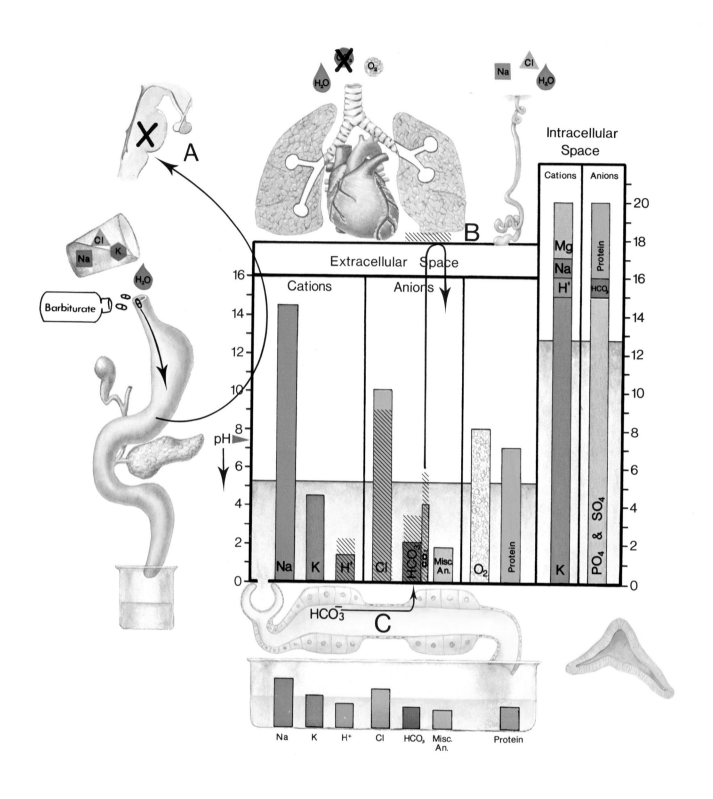

Summary of Abnormal Laboratory Findings

Serum H+—increased   Serum HCO₃⁻—   Blood pH—decreased
Serum Cl—decreased   increased   Blood Pco₂—increased

Barbiturate Intoxication

Pathophysiology

Ingestion of toxic amounts of barbiturates depresses the respiratory center (A). Thus *less carbon dioxide* is excreted via the lungs (B) and it *accumulates in the blood* with a corresponding *rise in* carbonic acid and *hydrogen ions*. Blood *pH drops*. The kidney compensates by reabsorbing more bicarbonate (C). Consequently the *serum bicarbonate rises*. The picture is similar to the respiratory acidosis of pulmonary emphysema (page 111).

Clinical Picture

Hypoventilation, lethargy and coma are the usual features. Deep tendon and corneal reflexes are present early, but may be absent in severe toxicity with coma.

Diagnosis

Blood and urine barbiturate levels will establish the diagnosis and differentiate this from other forms of respiratory acidosis.

Treatment

In mild toxicity, coffee by mouth or caffeine sodium benzoate intravenously may be all that is necessary. Of course lavage is done routinely regardless of the time between ingestion and discovery of the illness. Endotracheal intubation or tracheostomy may be necessary so that continuous IPPB may be given. Forced diuresis with 4 to 8 liters of 5 percent dextrose and saline or mannitol (Osmitrol 10-15%) is undertaken to rid the body of the barbiturate, provided that urine output is carefully monitored. Hypotension is treated with vasopressors (Aramine, etc.). Renal dialysis may be necessary in severe cases. Alkalinization of the blood may be useful in phenobarbital intoxication.

Etiology

Other central nervous system depressants, head trauma, and cerebrovascular disease may produce the same picture.

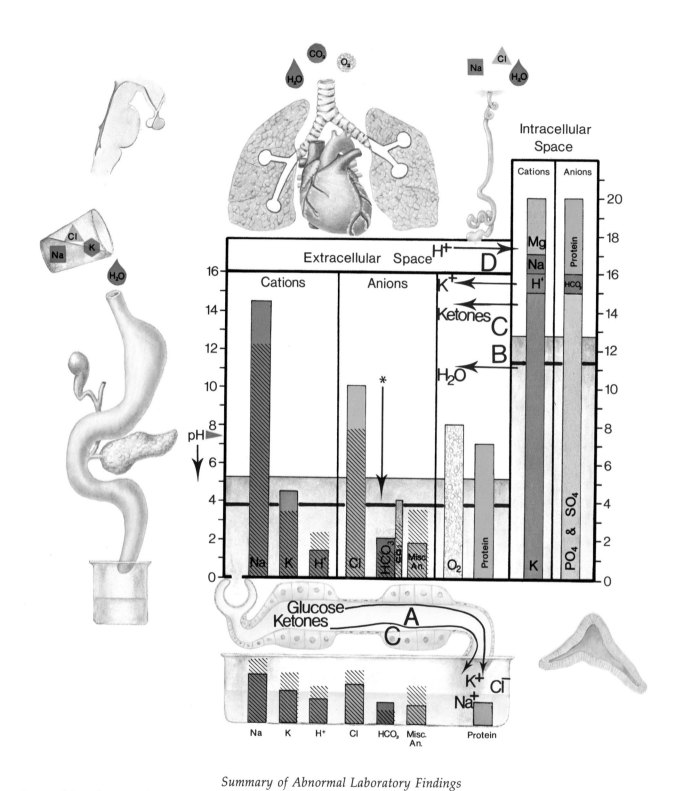

Summary of Abnormal Laboratory Findings

Serum Na—decreased
or normal
Serum K—decreased,
normal or increased
Serum H⁺—increased

Serum Cl—decreased or
normal
Serum HCO₃⁻—
decreased
Serum miscellaneous
anions—increased

Serum protein—
increased or normal
Blood volume—
decreased*
Blood pH—decreased

Blood P$_{CO_2}$—decreased
Urine volume—
decreased or normal
Urine Na—increased
Urine K—increased
Urine Cl—increased

Diabetic Ketoacidosis

Pathophysiology

In diabetic ketoacidosis the concentration of most of the serum electrolytes is reduced and body water is depleted. This eventuality follows a fascinating sequence of deviations from normal metabolism.

With an insufficient supply of insulin the cells are unable to utilize glucose in metabolism. The blood glucose rises and once it exceeds the renal threshold (170 mg.) spills into the urine and by its osmotic effect takes with it large amounts of water, sodium, chloride and potassium (A). *Serum sodium, potassium, chloride* and *blood volume decrease.* Intracellular water moves extracellularly in an attempt to maintain circulatory volume (B). Thus, *intracellular volume drops.* The cells must gain their energy from sources other than glucose. Therefore, large amounts of fat are mobilized and converted to ketones (C), such as acetoacetic acid and beta-hydroxybutyric acid, to meet this need. *Serum hydrogen ions increase.* These strong acids are neutralized by sodium bicarbonate and other buffers of the blood to form organic salts, water and carbon dioxide. *Serum bicarbonate drops.* Respirations are increased in order to blow off the carbon dioxide and increase blood pH. *Blood P_{CO_2} drops.* The *ketones* are utilized by the cells, but usually at a slower rate than their production so that their level *(miscellaneous anions) rises* in the blood and they spill into the urine taking with them sodium, potassium and water (C).

The kidney attempts to restore serum sodium bicarbonate by exchanging sodium for hydrogen ion and potassium and forming bicarbonate. However, its capacity to do this is limited.

Body potassium is lost by three additional mechanisms. First, potassium moves out of the cells (D) to replace serum sodium and in exchange for hydrogen ions to "buffer" the acidosis. Second, potassium is lost by cell catabolism for energy. Finally, lack of insulin blocks off an important avenue of potassium movement back into the cell. Despite these losses serum potassium is often normal or increased when the patient is first seen because of the hypovolemia and consequent impairment of renal function.

Clinical Picture

Hyperventilation, lethargy and coma along with signs of dehydration (page 77) are the usual findings. Many patients have vomiting and abdominal pain, so that an acute abdomen must be ruled out. A typical "fruity" odor (due to acetone) to the breath is noted in most cases.

Diagnosis

The serum electrolytes, pH, glucose and acetone are diagnostic in most cases. When the acetone is negative the lactic acid level should be ordered, since this may cause the coma in hypoxic states and in patients on phenformin.

Treatment

An infusion of isotonic saline is begun immediately after blood for sugar, acetone, electrolytes, BUN and gases are drawn. Regular insulin (one half the dose I.V. and one half subcutaneous) is given according to the plasma acetone as follows:

Acetone Still Positive at Plasma Dilution	Initial Dose of Insulin in Units
1:4	50
1:8	100
1:16	150
>1:16	200

Once the electrolytes are back, the bicarbonate deficit is calculated (formula on page 156) and sodium bicarbonate equal to one half the deficit is added to a solution of 0.45 percent hypotonic saline (not more than 44.6 mEq./500 ml.) and this is given. If the serum bicarbonate is above 12 mEq./L. it may be unnecessary to give any. If the potassium is low, 20 to 40 mEq. of potassium chloride are added to each bottle of 1,000 ml. of hypotonic saline after the deficit is calculated (formula on page 156). Three to four liters of fluid are usually required during the first four hours. If the blood sugar falls below 250 mg. the I.V. solution must be changed to 5 percent dextrose and one half normal saline with whatever other electrolyte deficits are required. Hypomagnesemia may develop and need attention.

Etiology

Undiagnosed diabetics and those who fail to take their insulin or suffer infection, trauma or surgical emergencies are particularly prone to develop this complication.

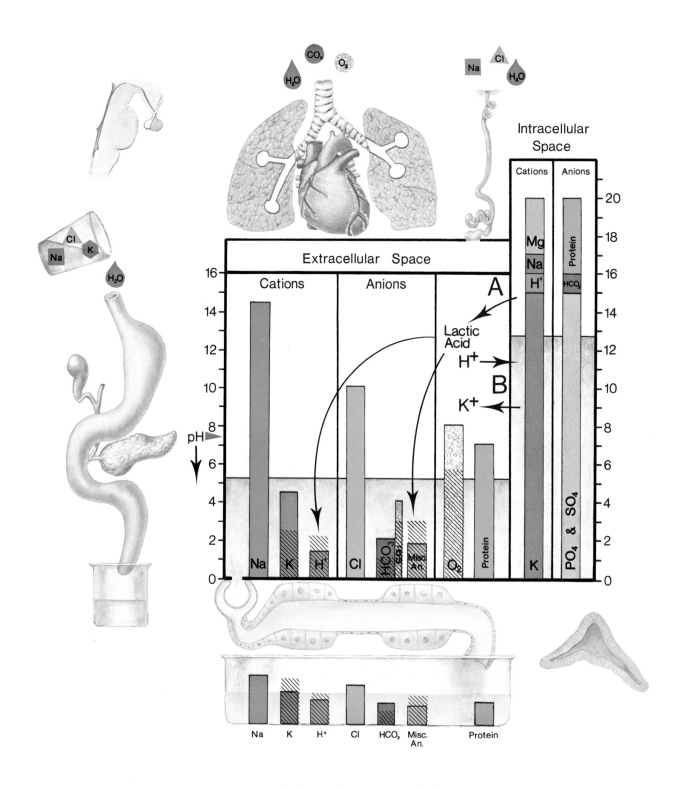

Summary of Abnormal Laboratory Findings

Serum Na—normal or decreased
Serum K—normal, decreased or increased
Serum H⁺—increased
Serum Cl—normal or decreased
Serum HCO₃⁻—decreased
Serum miscellaneous anions—increased
Blood pH—decreased
Blood Pco₂—decreased
Blood Po₂—decreased

Lactic Acidosis

Pathophysiology

Lactic acid is an end product of anaerobic glycolysis with each mole of glucose producing 2 moles of lactic acid. This is usually converted to pyruvic acid to enter the Krebs cycle where it is oxidized to carbon dioxide and water to produce energy. It may also be converted back to glucose by the liver for reserve energy. Lactic acid will accumulate whenever there is inadequate oxygen to convert it to pyruvate, or inadequate oxygen to oxidize pyruvate in the Kreb's cycle. It will also occur if the liver cannot convert it to glucose. The resulting lactic acidosis (A) causes a rise in *serum miscellaneous anions* and *hydrogen ions*. The *blood pH falls*. The buffers of the blood, particularly bicarbonate, neutralize the lactic acid and *serum bicarbonate falls* as it is converted to carbonic acid. The carbonic acid decomposes to carbon dioxide and water and the carbon dioxide is blown off by the lungs. Some of the hydrogen ions may shift into the cell in exchange for potassium (B). The kidney tries to compensate by exchanging more potassium and hydrogen ions for sodium in the tubules and forming more bicarbonate. Thus *potassium* is depleted and its *serum level may fall* if this mechanism for the "hydrogen ion exchange exceeds potassium" in the cells. Catabolism of cells for energy may also release more potassium as in diabetic ketoacidosis.

Clinical Picture

Hyperventilation, lethargy progressing to coma occurring in known diabetics or patients in shock or septicemia should make one suspect this condition. In contrast to ketoacidosis, there is no sweet odor to the breath and the condition develops in a matter of hours instead of two or three days.

Diagnosis

The history of diabetes or shock, the serum electrolytes, pH and blood gases illustrated plus the lack of ketonemia in the presence of a large, anion gap are significant diagnostic features. Blood lactate levels exceeding 7 mEq./L. (normal less than 1 mEq./L.) will pin down the diagnosis. If the patient has been on phenformin or alcohol, this condition should be strongly suspected.

Treatment

Most important in therapy is removal of the specific cause (sepis, shock, anoxia, phenformin, etc.). Restoring blood pressure to normal and administering oxygen may be lifesaving. The acidosis is treated like ketoacidosis except that bicarbonate deficits are corrected more swiftly and some bicarbonate is usually added to the initial infusions. From 200 to 400 mEq. or more of bicarbonate may have to be given in the first two to three hours. Blood gases should be done every half hour while correcting this deficit. Hemodialysis may be useful in removing both lactate and phenformin.[13]

Etiology

This condition may be induced in diabetics by phenformin administration, alcohol ingestion, shock, sepsis, pancreatitis or anything else that is associated with tissue hypoxia. In nondiabetics it is most frequently seen in cardiogenic or septic shock, but again anything that causes tissue hypoxia may be responsible.

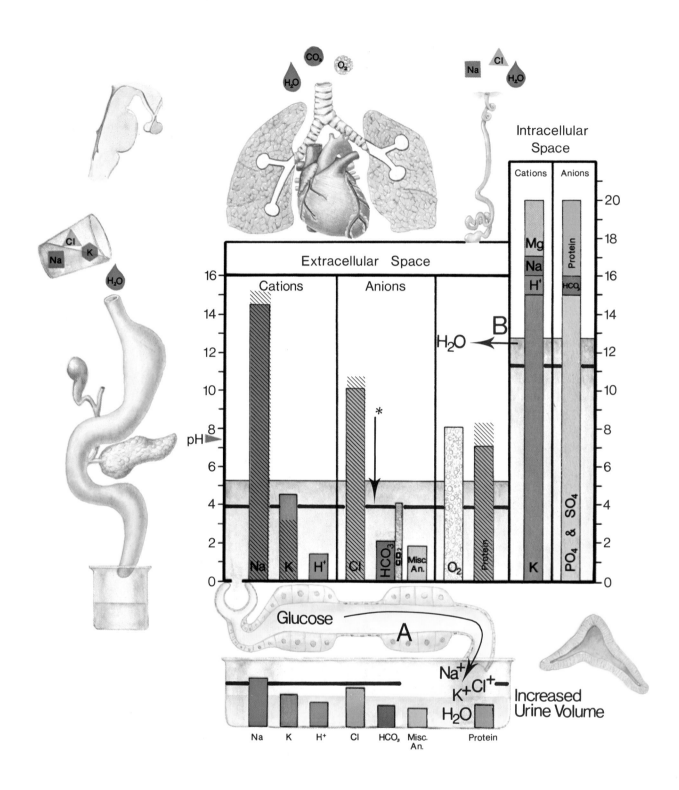

Summary of Abnormal Laboratory Findings

Serum Na—increased	Serum protein—
Serum K—decreased	increased
Serum Cl—increased	Blood volume—
Serum HCO₃⁻—normal	decreased*
or slightly decreased	

Hyperosmolar Nonketotic Diabetic Coma

Pathophysiology

Diabetics with this condition usually have normal or elevated plasma insulin levels. Thus they have enough insulin to prevent ketosis, but not enough to prevent hyperglycemia. The hyperglycemia leads to significant glycosuria (A) and a solute diuresis leading to severe dehydration and polyuria. Blood sugars of 4,800 mg. have been reported.[22] The hyperglycemia produces tremendous thirst causing these patients to drink water with more carbohydrate in it. Because of the diuresis, *plasma volume drops.* The diuresis takes with it significant amounts of sodium (50-60 mEq./L.). However *serum sodium* and *chloride* concentration *increases* because water is lost in excess of sodium. The resulting hyperosmolarity (which may be as high as 475 mOsm./L.) draws water from the cells (B) and *cell fluid volume decreases.* This leads to the neurologic features of this illness. Because of the prolonged diuresis, *serum potassium drops* as the kidney works to restore plasma volume by conserving sodium. Because there are no ketones the serum pH, hydrogen ion and bicarbonate usually do not change. However lactic acidosis has been reported to occur concomitantly.

Clinical Picture

A clouded sensorium, coma and even seizures are common. Focal neurologic signs are also seen. Fever is present in most cases but Kussmaul respirations are absent. Abdominal pain may result from the metabolic changes. Most of these patients are elderly.

Diagnosis

Plasma osmolality is the most important single test and it is always significantly elevated. It may be estimated roughly by the formula:

Plasma osmolality

$$= 2 \times \text{serum Na} + \frac{\text{Blood sugar}}{18}$$

Blood sugar values above 800 mg. are usual. The serum electrolytes are illustrated. The BUN is elevated. Hematocrit and *plasma protein* are *elevated* due to the loss of water. Blood volume is low. There is rarely ketonemia and only occasional ketonuria.

Treatment

Hypotonic saline and large insulin doses used to be considered the therapy of choice, but it has now been shown that correcting the sodium deficit and reexpanding the plasma volume is more important.[23] With large doses of insulin there is a rapid drop of blood glucose and without replacing it with sodium, shock and oliguria will result from the added drop in blood volume. Therefore isotonic saline and small doses of insulin (50-75 units in 24 hours) has been shown to be more prudent therapy. The calculated water deficit (using one half the plasma osmolality instead of the measured sodium in the formula on page 156) is administered over a 48-hour period or more unless there is an extreme emergency. This will prevent cerebral edema and water intoxication in the cells.

Etiology

Pancreatitis, severe burns, corticosteroids and diphenylhydantoin (Dilantin) therapy and peritoneal dialysis are among the many conditions that may precipitate this state.

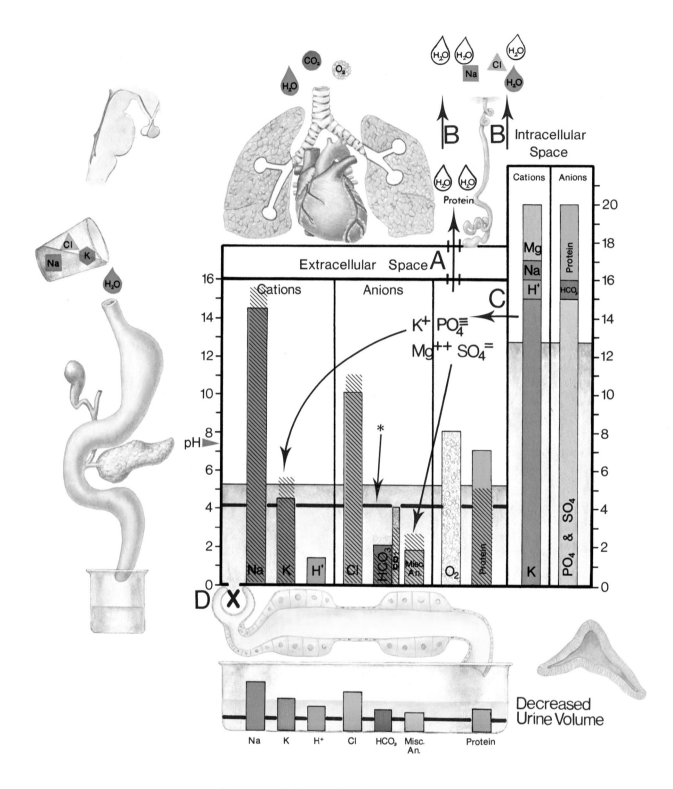

Summary of Abnormal Laboratory Findings
Serum Na—increased
Serum K—increased
Serum Cl—increased
Serum HCO$_3^-$—
    decreased

Serum Protein—
    decreased
Blood volume—
    decreased*
Urine volume—
    decreased

Second and Third Degree Burns

Pathophysiology

Patients with third degree burns suffer losses and imbalances of fluid and electrolytes by three mechanisms. First, damaged capillaries in the burned areas leak large quantities of plasmalike fluid into the burned areas (A). This *reduces plasma volume* considerably. Second, insensible water loss from the burned area increases from 10 to 20 times normal (B) leading to *hypernatremia* and *hyperchloremia*. Third, the damaged (burned) tissue leaks *potassium, magnesium,* and *miscellaneous anions* into the plasma and extracellular fluid (C). Serum *potassium* and *miscellaneous anions rise,* especially if there is decreased renal function (D) from the associated shock. The caloric and nutritional needs of the burned patient rise because it requires 560 Kcal. to evaporate each liter of water from the burned surface. Burned patients may lose 25 to 300 ml./sq. m. of burned body surface per hour.[4]

Clinical Picture

Aside from the changes in the burned areas there is often shock, hyperventilation and signs of dehydration. Urine output is usually decreased and anuria may develop from lower nephron nephrosis.

Diagnosis

The clinical picture and history establish the diagnosis in most cases. A determination of blood volume may indicate that the situation is more severe than the clinical appearance suggests.

Treatment

Aside from local treatment, fluid and electrolytes must be given in massive amounts. The rule of nines established by E. J. Pulaski and W. C. Tennison provides a rapid means of estimating the extent of the burns. The percentage of surface area occupied by each part of the body is as follows:

Head and neck—9%
Each upper extremity—9%
Front of trunk—18%
Back of trunk—18%
Each lower extremity—18%
Perineum—1%

Using the above method to establish the percentage of the body burned, the following (Brooke Army Formula) is used to determine the fluid requirements for the first 24 hours:

1. Plasma or colloid = 0.5 ml. × % burn × body wt. in Kg.
2. Electrolyte (lactated Ringer's) = 1.5 ml. × % burn × body wt. in Kg.
3. Basic needs = 5% dextrose and water (2,000 ml. for adults).

Burns of more than 50 percent of body surface are calculated as 50 percent.

Half of the fluid is infused in the first 8 hours, one quarter in the second 8 hours and one quarter in the third 8 hours, alternating the colloid with the electrolyte and followed by 5 percent dextrose and water in each eight-hour period. Blood replaces one fourth of the colloid when the hemoglobin is below 10.0 gm.

For the second 24-hour period, the plasma or colloid and Ringer's lactate are reduced to one half the amount calculated in the formula although the basic needs remain the same. During the third 24-hour period only the basic needs (2,000 ml. of 5% dextrose/water) are given, because edema fluid in the burn begins to return to the circulation and brings sufficient electrolytes with it.

This is only one of the formulas for burn therapy but it has stood the test of time. However, no formula can be followed routinely and the rate of infusion must be in accord with the clinical reaction of the patient.

Etiology

Fire, gasoline and chemical burns of all types may necessitate the same treatment.

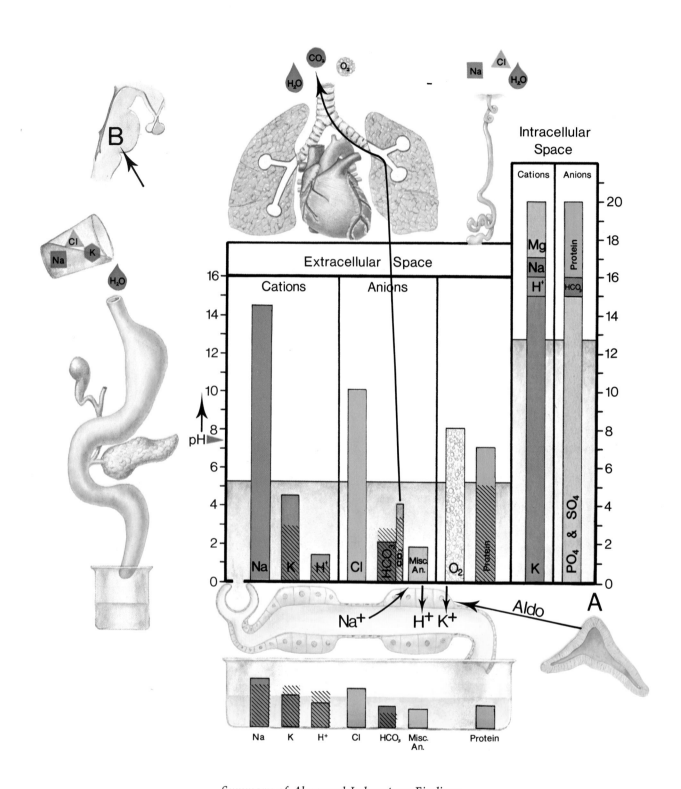

Summary of Abnormal Laboratory Findings

Serum K—decreased or normal

Serum H⁺—decreased or normal

Serum HCO₃⁻—normal or increased

Serum protein—decreased

Blood volume—normal or increased

Blood pH—increased

Blood Pco₂—decreased

Cirrhosis of the Liver with Ascites

Pathophysiology

In this disorder there is a *decreased production* of *plasma proteins*, especially albumin, with a consequent decrease in "effective" plasma volume and renal plasma flow. This leads to an activation of the renin-angiotensin system and secretion of aldosterone (secondary aldosteronism) (A). More sodium is reabsorbed from the distal tubule in exchange for hydrogen ions and potassium. Thus there is a temporary increase in serum sodium and a *decrease* in *serum potassium* and *hydrogen ion* with a mild metabolic alkalosis. However the sodium retains water with it and while there is a net gain in total body water and sodium the serum sodium is not increased in most of these subjects.[2] Both plasma and urine aldosterone levels are greatly increased.[24] Despite the *decreased serum total proteins and decreased "effective" plasma volume*, total plasma volume is normal or increased possibly because of the expanded volume in the obstructed portal veins. Serum bicarbonate does not usually increase, since there is an associated mild respiratory alkalosis due to stimulation of the respiratory center by hyperammonemia (B). *Blood pH* is nevertheless *increased* in both types of alkalosis.

Clinical Picture

An enlarged, hard, nodular liver, ascites, spider angiomata, liver palms, distended superficial abdominal veins, hemorrhoids and mild jaundice are the usual findings. The patient's sensorium may be clouded. There may be edema of the lower extremities and generalized emaciation.

Diagnosis

The electrolyte picture is not diagnostic, but the clinical findings together with abnormal liver function tests (BSP, transaminase, alkaline phosphates, etc.) and a liver biopsy establish the diagnosis. In patients with severe jaundice, obstruction of the biliary tree can be ruled out by an excretion liver scan or transhepatic cholangiography and endoscopic retrograde cholangiography.

Treatment

In the early stages thiazide diuretics combined with spironolactone (aldosterone antagonist) and a moderate to high protein diet may control the situation. Stronger diuretics (furosemide, etc.) and salt-free albumin may be necessary to control the edema and ascites, but one should remember that these drugs may precipitate hepatic coma. Therapeutic paracentesis is indicated only in rare circumstances.

Etiology

Alcoholic cirrhoisis, viral hepatitis with postnecrotic cirrhosis and carcinoma of the liver may cause this picture.

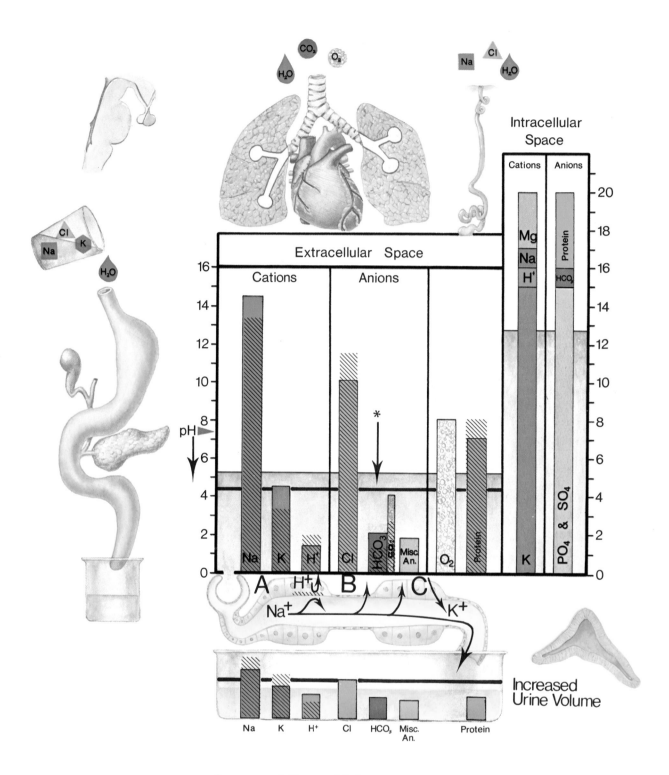

Summary of Abnormal Laboratory Findings

Serum Na—decreased
Serum K—decreased
Serum H+—increased
Serum Cl—increased
Serum HCO₃⁻—
    decreased

Blood volume—
    decreased*
Blood pH—decreased
Urine volume—
    increased

Acetazolamide Diuretics

Pathophysiology

This diuretic inhibits carbonic anhydrase activity in the proximal tubule (A), thus blocking the exchange of hydrogen ion for sodium there. The following illustrations depict this change:

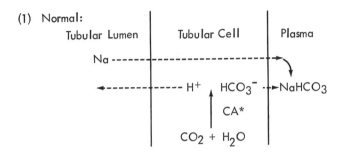

(1) Normal:

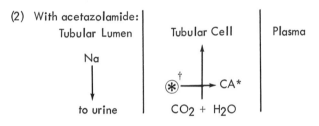

(2) With acetazolamide:

*CA = Carbonic Anhydrase
† ⊛ = Inhibition

Hydrogen ions are retained and their serum level *rises* while *pH drops.* Serum *bicarbonate drops* along with *sodium* because less is formed.

However, while 60 percent of filtered sodium is inhibited from reabsorption at this site the sodium moves on to the ascending limb of Henle where much of it is absorbed almost exclusively with chloride (B). Thus there is *hyperchloremia* with a metabolic acidosis. The rest of the sodium moves on to the distal tubule. Because reabsorption of sodium is inhibited in the proximal tubule a greater burden is put on the distal tubule to reabsorb sodium in exchange for potassium (C). Thus *hypokalemia develops.* The net loss of sodium is only 2 to 3 percent of the glomerular filtrate.[25] Consequently this diuretic is most useful in combination with diuretics that act on the loop of Henle or distal tubule.

Clinical Picture

The patient usually has no unusual symptoms on this therapy. However, large doses may cause drowsiness and paresthesias. Since the drug is related to the sulfonamides, hypersensitivity reactions are not uncommon.

Diagnosis

The serum electrolytes, arterial blood gases and history of drug ingestion usually establish the diagnosis.

Treatment

Withholding the drug is usually all that is necessary, but potassium and sodium bicarbonate may have to be given in severe toxicity.

Etiology

The electrolyte changes are similar to those of renal tubular acidosis and ammonium chloride administration.

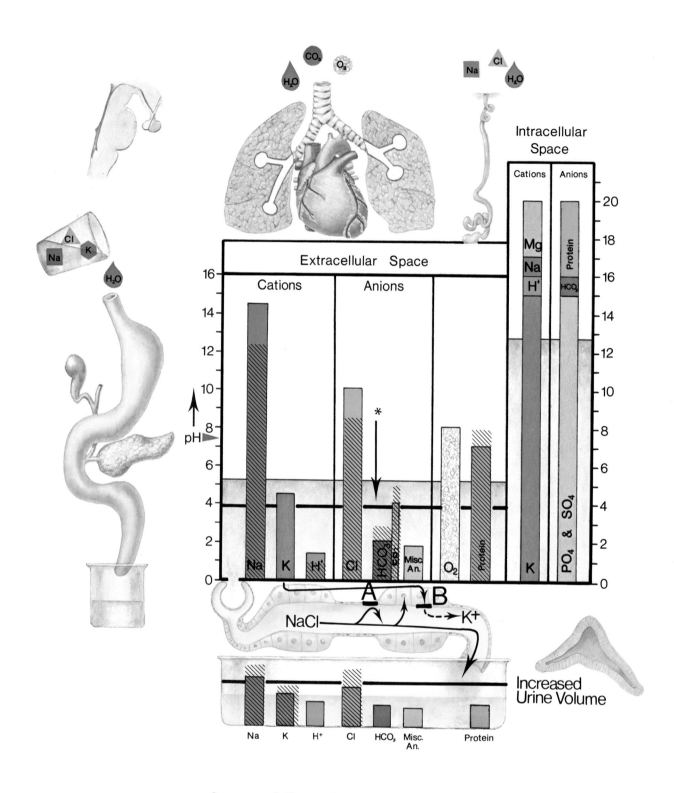

Summary of Abnormal Laboratory Findings

Serum Na—decreased
Serum K—decreased or
    normal
Serum H⁺—decreased
Serum Cl—decreased

Serum HCO₃⁻—
    increased
Blood volume—
    decreased*
Blood pH—increased

Urine Na—increased
Urine Cl—increased
Urine K—increased
Urine volume—
    increased

Mercurial Diuretics

Pathophysiology

Like furosemide and ethacrynic acid these diuretics inhibit sodium and chloride reabsorption in the ascending limb of Henle (A). *Serum sodium and chloride drop.* The unabsorbed sodium is passed on to the distal tubule where it might all be reabsorbed in exchange for potassium were it not for the fact that these drugs probably inhibit potassium secretion too (B). However, this inhibition is only partial so that *hypokalemia* may develop with continued use of these diuretics just as it does in other diuretic therapy. Reabsorption of sodium bicarbonate in the proximal tubule is uninhibited so that *serum bicarbonate increases* to make up the deficit in anions from the chloride loss. Thus a hypochloremic metabolic alkalosis results.

Clinical Picture

Most patients experience no side effects while on these diuretics. However, signs of dehydration (page 77) and hypokalemia (page 39) may develop with continued use. Acute tubular necrosis and hypersensitivity reactions may occur in some patients.

Diagnosis

The serum electrolytes coupled with the history of administration of this drug usually establishes the diagnosis. Aldosteronism, pyloric obstruction and other causes of a metabolic alkalosis may have to be considered in doubtful cases.

Treatment

Withholding the drug is usually all that is necessary when the hypokalemia and alkalosis are mild. A liter of isotonic saline with 20 to 30 mEq. of potassium chloride added may be given intravenously in acute cases.

Etiology

This is discussed under pathophysiology.

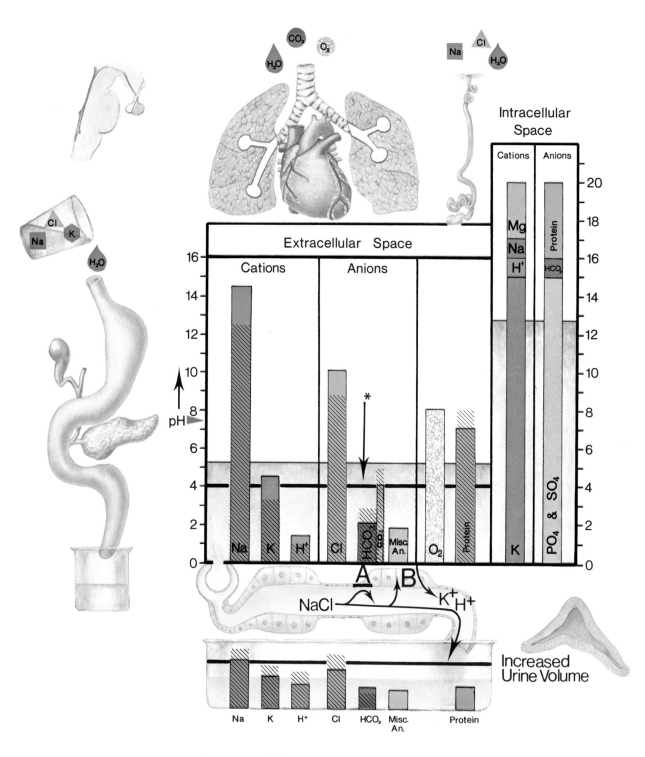

Summary of Abnormal Laboratory Findings

Serum Na—decreased
Serum K—decreased
Serum H⁺—decreased
  or normal
Serum Cl—decreased
Serum HCO₃⁻—
  increased or normal

Serum protein—
  increased
Blood volume—
  decreased (rarely
  increased)*

Blood pH—increased or
  normal
Urine volume—
  increased
Urine Na—increased
Urine K—increased
Urine Cl—increased

Thiazide Diuretics

Pathophysiology

These drugs inhibit selective reabsorption of sodium and chloride in the early distal tubule (A) where tubular fluid is being rendered hypotonic.[26] Thus *serum sodium* and *chloride fall*. The sodium remaining in the tubular lumen is delivered to the main portion of the distal tubule where an increased burden is placed on the "H^+ for Na^+" and the "K^+ for Na^+ exchange" (B). Thus many patients on these drugs have *hypokalemia* and a metabolic alkalosis with *decreased serum hydrogen ion* and *increased serum bicarbonate*. Because these drugs exert slight inhibition of carbonic anhydrase[2] the metabolic alkalosis is not as severe as with mercurial diuretics.

Clinical Picture

Signs of dehydration (page 77) hypokalemia (page 39) and clinical gout due to hyperuricemia may occur. These drugs are diabetogenic like furosemide, but this is mild. More important they may aggravate a dilutional hyponatremia because they cause inappropriate secretion of ADH.[27] A small number of patients may develop hypercalcemia. Hypersensitivity reactions occur as these drugs are related to sulfonamide.

Diagnosis

The finding of a hypokalemic metabolic alkalosis in a patient on thiazide diuretics usually establishes the diagnosis. Primary and secondary aldosteronism must be considered, but the low sodium will usually rule out the former. Dilutional hyponatremia may be ruled out by measuring the CVP, blood volume, and serum protein.

Treatment

Withholding the drug is usually all that is necessary. It is wise to give a potassium supplement of at least 30 to 40 mEq./day to patients on these drugs. A 10 percent solution of potassium chloride is best for this purpose. An aldosterone antagonist (spironolactone) may be used to spare potassium also. Benemid can be administered concomitantly to control the hyperuricemia. Occasionally isotonic or hypertonic saline must be given to control severe hyponatremia and dehydration.

Etiology

All the benzothiadiazines, phthalimidines (Hygroton) and quinazolinones produce a similar picture.

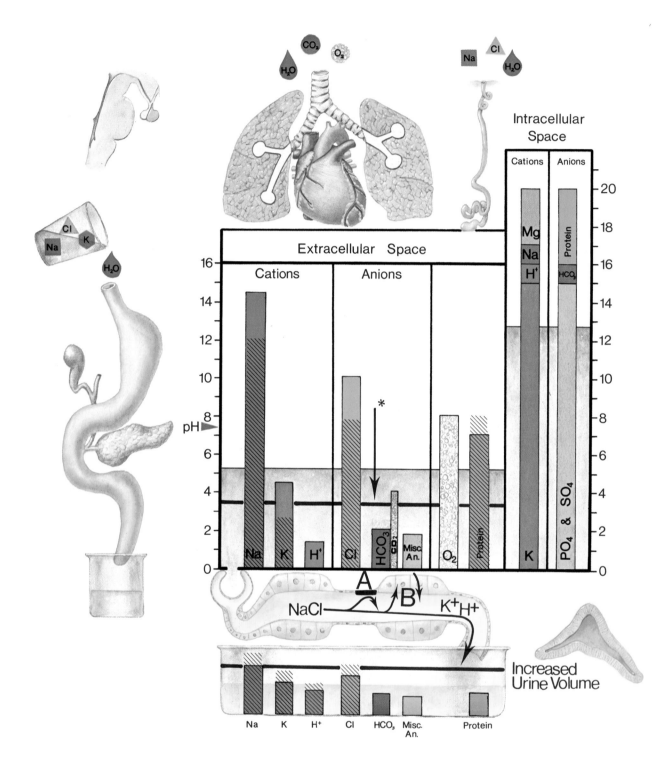

Summary of Abnormal Laboratory Findings

Serum Na—decreased   Blood volume—
Serum K—decreased   decreased*
Serum Cl—decreased   Urine volume—
Serum HCO₃⁻—normal   increased
  or increased   Urine Na—increased
Serum protein—   Urine K—increased
  increased   Urine Cl—increased

Furosemide and Ethacrynic Acid Diuretics

Pathophysiology

Both of these diuretics inhibit sodium reabsorption with chloride in the ascending limb of Henle (A). Thus *serum sodium and chloride and plasma volume drop.* As much as 25 percent of the sodium passing through the glomerular filtration is excreted in patients on these diuretics so they are obviously very potent. Some of the sodium blocked from reabsorption in the ascending limb of Henle is reabsorbed in exchange for hydrogen ion and potassium in the distal tubule (B). Thus *serum potassium decreases* and there may occasionally be a metabolic alkalosis from increased hydrogen ion excretion. Unlike acetazolamide these diuretics do not produce any consistent alteration in acid-base balance.

Clinical Picture

Since these drugs can produce a massive diuresis, dehydration may develop rather rapidly. The plasma and extracellular volume may contract so drastically that shock and prerenal azotemia develop. Hyperuricemia, hyperglycemia (with furosemide), vertigo, tinnitus and deafness (rare) may develop. Some patients develop clinical gout. Signs of hypokalemia (page 39) are frequent when patients are not given supplemental potassium or followed often enough.

Hypersensitivity reactions may occur (especially with furosemide because it is related to sulfonamide).

Diagnosis

The serum electrolyte and history of diuretic therapy with these agents are usually sufficient to establish the diagnosis. However differentiation from dilutional hyponatremia may be difficult. Blood volume studies, central venous pressure evaluation, serum protein, hematocrit and a spinal tap (which shows a low pressure in hyponatremia from diuretics) are all helpful in distinguishing between the two.

Treatment

In most cases of toxicity, withholding the drug is all that is necessary. If the serum sodium is below 115 mEq./L. or there is shock, hypertonic saline (3-5%) and potassium should be given intravenously, but not more than 1 to 2 ml./min. It is not wise to raise the serum sodium more than 10 mEq. in 24 hours.

Etiology

Discussed under pathophysiology.

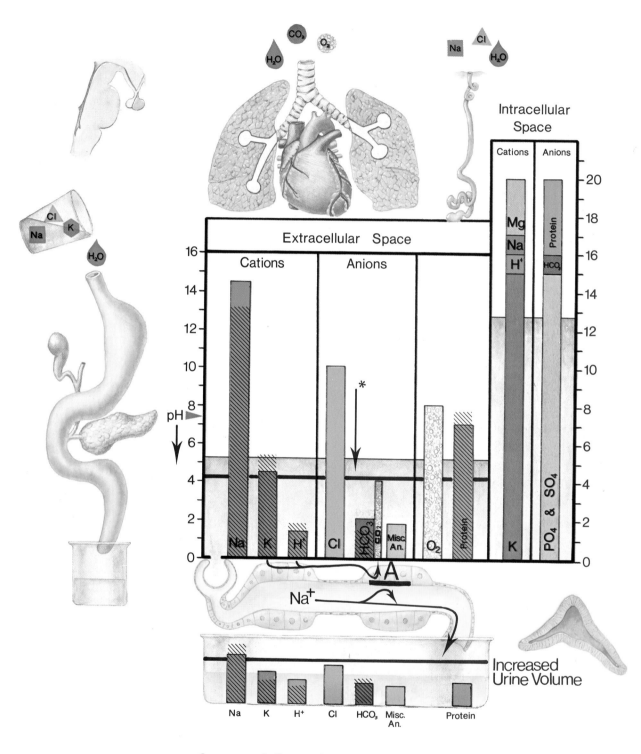

Summary of Abnormal Laboratory Findings

Serum Na—decreased
Serum K—increased
Serum H⁺ ion—
    increased
Serum HCO₃⁻—
    decreased

Blood volume—
    decreased*
Urine volume—
    increased
Urine Na—increased

Spironolactone

Pathophysiology

This drug antagonizes the action of aldosterone on the distal tubule. Thus sodium is not reabsorbed in exchange for hydrogen ion and potassium (A) so that *serum sodium drops* slightly and *serum hydrogen ion and potassium rise.* Since it is a weak diuretic it is usually given in combination with other diuretics. However in patients with secondary aldosteronism (cirrhotics, nephrotics, etc.) it is very useful.

Clinical Picture

Lethargy and weakness may develop from the metabolic acidosis and hyperkalemia. The hyperkalemia may also induce cardiac arrhythmias. Hyponatremic dehydration is unusual. Since this drug is structurally related to progesterone, it may cause hirsutism, gynecomastia and gastrointestinal distress. Reversible azotemia may also develop.

Diagnosis

The hyperkalemic metabolic acidosis together with a history of using this drug usually establishes the diagnosis.

Treatment

Withholding the drug is usually sufficient for treating toxicity, but intravenous 50 percent dextrose and insulin, calcium gluconate or sodium bicarbonate may be necessary in acute hyperkalemia with cardiac arrhythmias. Cation exchange resins (Kayexalate) may be given by mouth or by enema in less acute hyperkalemia.

Etiology

Triamterene (Dyrenium) may cause the same picture by its action on the distal tubule and collecting ducts, but it is not an aldosterone antagonist.

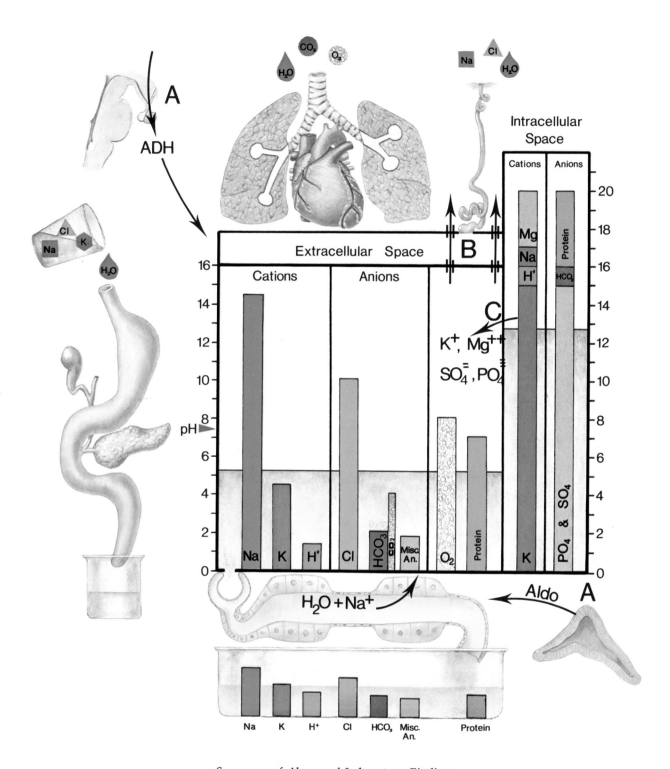

Summary of Abnormal Laboratory Findings

Serum Na—normal or
  increased
Serum K—normal or
  decreased
Serum H+ ion—normal
  or decreased

Serum Cl—normal
Serum HCO₃⁻—normal
  or increased
Blood volume—normal
  or decreased

Surgery and Trauma

Pathophysiology

The daily fluid and electrolyte losses of a healthy adult are between 1,800 and 2,000 ml. of water, 70 to 80 mEq. of sodium chloride and 40 to 60 mEq. of potassium. During surgery and trauma, either due to a decrease in effective plasma volume or from the effects of anesthesia on the hypothalamus and adrenal cortex, there is increased secretion of aldosterone, glucocorticoids and ADH (A). Consequently the kidneys retain sodium and water. Serum sodium does not usually rise because of the water retention. During major surgery 150 to 200 ml. of a plasmalike fluid is lost into the operative site (B) for each hour of the procedure. This must be replaced. Surgical and nonsurgical trauma lead to cell breakdown and release of potassium, magnesium and miscellaneous anions (C). Nevertheless, the level of these electrolytes does not rise unless there is shock or renal failure.

Clinical Picture

This will be related to the underlying condition, but shock, infection and other complications must be anticipated.

Diagnosis

Since the serum electrolytes are often normal, the diagnosis of electrolyte imbalances during and after surgery and trauma will depend more on daily weighing of the patient and observing urine output and losses from nasogastric suction, sweat, increased respiration and wound drains. If the picture is complicated by an underlying disease such as diabetes, congestive heart failure and renal failure, careful observation to see that these are controlled may be more important.

Treatment

Day of Surgery or Trauma. Since sodium is retained, no sodium is given. In procedures lasting one or two hours (cholecystectomy, hysterectomy), only 200 to 500 ml. of a balanced electrolyte formula would be lost from the operative site and much of this is replaced by electrolytes from injured tissue. The usual prescription for the day is:

> 2,000 ml. of 5% dextrose and water with 20 mEq. of KCl added to each bottle of 1000 ml. This is given at 125 to 150 ml./hour.

First Postoperative Day. The prescription is the same as for the day of surgery except that losses from nasogastric suction or other drainage sites are added and given as one-half normal saline with 20 mEq. of KCl/L. for gastric juice and Ringer's lactate with 15 mEq./KCl added to each liter for intestinal, biliary and pancreatic juices. Urine output should be at least 1,000 ml. a day. If it is not, a central venous pressure catheter is put in and if it does not show an elevated venous pressure, fluids of the type already outlined are increased until either CVP rises above 15 cm. or urine output is increased to 50 ml./hour. If urine output remains low see Acute Renal Failure page 107.

Second Postoperative Day. By now the body's tendency to retain sodium is reduced and urine output should be stabilized. A good prescription would be 2,000 to 3,000 ml. of 5 percent dextrose and 0.3 normal saline with 20 mEq. of KCl added to each liter. Losses from nasogastric suction and drains are added to this as in the first postoperative day.

Etiology

The title is self-explanatory.

Section Five
Fluid and Electrolyte Therapy

Fluid and electrolyte therapy involves the replacement of deficits, supplying daily maintenance requirements, and replacing continued losses.

Formulas for Calculating Fluid and Electrolyte Deficits

Water

$$\text{Body water deficit} = \text{normal body water} - \text{current body water}$$

Since normal body weight is usually known, normal body water may be calculated by:

$$\text{Normal body water} = 0.6 \times \text{normal body wt. in Kg.}$$

Current body water is not known, but may be calculated by the following formulas:

$$\text{Current body water} = \frac{\text{ideal serum Na} \times \text{normal body water}}{\text{measured serum Na}}$$

Thus:

$$\text{Body water deficit} = 0.6 \times \text{normal body wt. (Kg.)} - \frac{(\text{ideal serum Na} \times 0.6 \times \text{normal body wt.})}{(\text{measured serum Na})}$$

Ideal serum Na for this formula is 138 mEq./L.

For example: A 60-Kg. male has a serum sodium of 158 mEq./L. What is his body water deficit?

$$\text{Body water deficit} = 0.6 \times 60 - \frac{(138 \times .6 \times 60)}{158}$$
$$\text{Body water deficit} = 36 - \frac{(138 \times 36)}{158}$$
$$\text{Body water deficit} = 36 - 31.5$$
$$\text{Body water deficit} = 4.5 \text{ liters}$$

A simpler formula can be developed on the following principle: The percentage decrease in body water will be proportional to the percentage increase in serum sodium.
Thus:

$$\text{Body water deficit} = \frac{\text{measured Na} - \text{ideal Na}}{\text{ideal Na}} \times \text{normal body water}$$

In the 60-Kg. male used in the example above the deficit would be calculated:

$$\text{Body water deficit} = \frac{158 - 138}{138} \times 36$$
$$\text{Body water deficit} = \frac{20}{138} \times 36 = 5.2 \text{ liters}$$

Some patients with dehydration have a normal sodium and this formula will not be helpful. Blood volume and CVP must be used to monitor fluid replacement under these circumstances.

Sodium. Since most of the sodium is in the extracellular fluid, the sodium deficit will be the difference between the ideal serum sodium and the measured serum sodium multiplied by the number of liters of fluid in the extracellular fluid. The extracellular fluid is roughly 20 percent of the body weight. The following formula is used:

$$\text{Sodium deficit} = \text{ideal serum sodium} - \text{measured serum sodium} \times .20 \times \text{body wt. in Kg.}$$

For example, a 70-Kg. male has a serum sodium of 120 mEq./L.

$$\text{Sodium deficit} = 138 \text{ (ideal serum Na)} - 120 \times .20 \times 70 \text{ Kg.}$$
$$\text{Sodium deficit} = 138 - 120 \times 14$$
$$= 252 \text{ mEq.}$$

Potassium. To replace the potassium in the extracellular fluid we could use a formula similar to the one for sodium deficits, but since most of the potassium is intracellular we want to replace the loss in a volume at least twice the extracellular fluid. The following formula is used:

$$\text{Potassium deficit} = \text{ideal potassium} - \text{measured potassium} \times .40 \times \text{body wt. in Kg.}$$

For example, in a 60-Kg. female with a potassium of 2.0 mEq./L. how many mEq. are needed?

$$\text{Potassium deficit} = 4.5 \text{ (ideal K)} - 2.0 \times .40 \times 60$$
$$\text{Potassium deficit} = 2.5 \times 24$$
$$\text{Potassium deficit} = 60 \text{ mEq.}$$

Bicarbonate. Most of the body bicarbonate exists in the extracellular fluid so that a formula similar to that used in calculating sodium deficits could be used if it were not for two things. There is some intracellular bicarbonate. Furthermore, other buffers of the extracellular and intracellular fluid must be relieved of their hydrogen ion to restore acid-base balance. For this reason a volume double the extracellular fluid is used in the formula as follows:

$$HCO_3^- \text{ deficit} = \text{ideal } HCO_3^- - \text{measured } HCO_3^- \times 0.4 \times \text{body wt. in Kg.}$$

For example, a 55-Kg. female had a bicarbonate of 10 mEq./L. What is her deficit?

$$HCO_3^- \text{ deficit} = 25 \text{ (ideal } HCO_3^-) - 10$$
$$\times 0.4 \times 55$$
$$HCO_3^- \text{ deficit} = 15 \times 0.4 \times 55$$
$$HCO_3^- \text{ deficit} = 330 \text{ mEq.}$$

Chloride. With serum chlorides above 90 mEq. no deficit need be replaced. Below that a formula similar to that used in sodium deficits may be used since most of the body chloride lies in the extracellular fluid.
Thus:

$$\text{Chloride deficit} = \text{ideal chloride (100)}$$
$$- \text{ measured chloride}$$
$$\times 0.2 \times \text{body wt. in Kg.}$$

Summary. These are the major formulas used in fluid and electrolyte therapy of adults. They are not exact so that most clinicians give half of the calculated deficit in two to six hours and then reevaluate the situation, except in life-threatening emergencies.

Maintenance Requirements

In previous chapters the basic daily needs for water, sodium chloride and potassium have been discussed. These may be summarized as follows:[28]

Water: 1,800 ml.
NaCl: 70 – 80 mEq.
Potassium: 40 – 60 mEq.

In addition, the body needs 600 to 800 calories daily to avoid the catabolism of fat and protein for energy and prevent a metabolic acidosis. This is supplied as 150 to 200 gm. of glucose. Therefore a suitable prescription for daily maintenance requirements would be:

1. 1,500 ml. of 10 percent dextrose and water
2. 500 ml. of 5 percent dextrose and normal saline.

3. 50 mEq. of KCl, 20 of which could be added to the first 1,000 ml. of 10 percent dextrose and water, 10 to the next 500 ml. of 10 percent dextrose and water, and 20 to the 500 ml. of 5 percent dextrose and normal saline.

In addition some authorities[14] add 1 to 2 ml. of 50 percent $MgSO_4 \cdot 7H_2O$.

This prescription would of course have to be modified according to the urine output, rate of respirations, sweating, age and weight of the individual in question.

Remember, too rapid administration of glucose solutions may cause a solute diuresis and a significant water deficit can result. Therefore, the fluid should be administered over not less than a 10- or 12-hour period (150-200 ml./hour).

Replacement of Continued Losses

In addition to maintenance requirements and replacement of calculated deficits at the time he first sees the patient, the clinician must keep a daily record of losses through nasogastric suction, drainage sites, diarrhea, sweat and excessive urine output and replace them. Table 6 shows the average composition of fluid and electrolytes in the various body fluids together with the most appropriate solutions for their replacement. Most replacement of losses can be done with the following solutions:

5% Dextrose and water
One-half normal Saline
5% Dextrose and one-half normal saline
20-ml. Ampules of 14.9% KCl (40 mEq./amp.)
50-ml. Ampules of 7.5% $NaHCO_3$ (44.6 mEq./amp.)

One need only use Table 6 to determine the deficit and mix the five solutions above appropriately.

In Table 7 are listed the thirteen major electrolyte solutions that will cover the needs of almost all clinical situations. Reference is made to these solutions in the treatment of specific clinical disorders throughout this text. Copies of these two tables or similar tables should be kept with the clinician at all times.

TABLE 6. Fluid and Electrolyte Composition of Body Fluids

FLUID	WATER in ml.	Na mEq./L.	K mEq./L.	H⁺	pH	Cl mEq./L.	HCO₃⁻ mEq./L.	REPLACEMENT FLUID
Blood	7% body wt. in Kg.	138	4.5		7.35-7.45	103	25	Blood, saline, plasma, Dextran
Extracellular	20% of body wt. in Kg.	145	4.0		7.35-7.45	115	27	Lactated Ringer's solution
Intracellular	60% of body wt. in Kg.	10	150			5	10	Nothing suitable, but Isolyte P and Isolyte M the best
Urine	800-1,500/day	30-80	30-80		5-7	50-100		5% Dextrose and normal saline with 20-30 mEq. KCl/L.
Sweat	0-2400/day	50	5			55		N/3 saline and 5% dextrose
Gastric (Adults)	2500/day	20-100	5-25	90	1-7	90-155		N/2 saline with 20 mEq. KCl/L.
Bile	500/day	120-150	3-12		7-8	80-120	30-50	Ringer's lactate with 15 mEq. of KCl/L.
Pancreatic	700/day	110-150	3-10		7-8	40-80	70-110	N/2 saline with 2 amps. NaHCO₃ and 20 mEq. KCl each liter
Small Intestine	3000/day	80-150	2-10			90-131	20-40	Ringer's lactate with 15 mEq. KCl for each liter
Normal Stool	100/day	5 mEq./day	10 mEq./day			10 mEq./day		None necessary when volume below 100 ml. a day
Expiratory Air (insensible loss)	600-800/day							5% D & W (especially in hyperventilation)
Skin (insensible loss)	100-200/day							5% D & W (especially in fever)
Diarrhea (Adults)	6,000-10,000/day	50	45		7-8	115	29	1. Isolyte M with 5% dextrose 2. .45% hypotonic saline with 40 mEq. KCl and 1/2 amp. NaHCO₃
Intestinal Suction	1,000-5,000/day	130	20		7-8	115	29	1. Lactated potassic saline solution (Darrow's)
Gastric (infants) <12 Kg.	1,000-2,500/day	75	20			100		N/2 saline and 20 mEq. KCl/L.
Diarrhea (infants) <12 Kg.	1,000-2,500/day	60	30			45	29	Inosol B with 5% dextrose

TABLE 7. Major Electrolyte Composition of Recommended Fluids and Their Uses

SOLUTION	Na mEq./L.	K mEq./L.	Cl mEq./L.	HCO$_3^-$ mEq./L.	Glucose gm./L.	PRINCIPAL USES
5% Dextrose and Water					50	Insensible water loss Dehydration (hypertonic) First day postoperative
10% Dextrose and Water					100	Dehydration Block protein catabolism Parenteral alimentation
2½% Dextrose and Water					25	Pediatric dehydration
Normal (isotonic) Saline	154		154			Hyponatremia Replacement of ECF
5% Dextrose and Normal Saline	154		154		50	Part of daily maintenance formula May be used when rapid replacement of sodium and caloric deficit needed
N/2 Saline	77		77			Good basic solution for replacement prescription
N/2 Saline and 5% Dextrose	77		77		50	Best maintenance solution (with KCl added)
N/4 Saline and 5% Dextrose	38		38		50	Pediatric maintenance and basic replacement solution for infants
3% Hypertonic Saline	513		513			Correction of symptomatic sodium deficit
14.9% KCl (20 ml./amp.)		40/amp.	40/amp.			Additive to other solution for daily maintenance and replacement of losses. Treatment of metabolic alkalosis and acidosis
7.5% NaHCO$_3$	44.6/amp.			44.6/amp.		Additive for replacement of G.I. losses Treatment of metabolic acidosis
Lactated Ringer's Solution (Hartman's)	130	4	112	28		Best solution for replacement of ECF volume and fluid losses from operative site and intestinal obstruction and burns
Lactated Potassic Saline Solution (Darrow's)	121	35	103	53		Losses in diarrhea and biliary or intestinal fistulas

TABLE 8. Nomogram for Determination of Body Surface Area from Height and Weight[1]

Height	Surface Area	Weight
feet centimetres	square metres	pounds kilograms

[1]From the formula of DuBois and DuBois, *Arch. Intern. Med.*, 17:863, 1916: $S = W^{0.425} \times H^{0.725} \times 71.84$, or: $\log S = 0.425 \log W + 0.725 \log H + 1.8564$. ($S$ = body surface in square centimetres, W = weight in kilograms, H = height in centimetres.)

Section Six
Diagnostic and Treatment Problems

DIAGNOSTIC PROBLEMS

Diagnostic Problems—Case 1

O.B., is a 51-year-old semiconscious white male whose admission electrolytes were:

Na—138 mEq./L.
K—3.5 mEq./L.
Cl—74 mEq./L.
HCO_3^-—56 mEq./L.

A look at Table 2 fails to show a pattern with a normal sodium, low normal potassium, low chloride and high bicarbonate. Table 4 shows a laboratory error, pulmonary emphysema, aldosteronism and pyloric obstruction to be the most likely possibilities. A laboratory error can be almost eliminated because the anion gap was normal:

Anion gap = $(Na + K) - (Cl + HCO_3^-)$
Anion gap = $(138 + 3.5) - (74 + 56)$
Anion gap = 11.5 (normal = 12 ± 4)

Indeed repeat electrolytes done by the laboratory yielded the same results.

The most striking abnormalities here are the low chloride and high bicarbonate. Table 1 shows three common conditions that have these abnormalities: pulmonary emphysema, primary aldosteronism and pyloric obstruction. Clinical examination revealed no history or physical findings of pulmonary emphysema so that this is pretty well ruled out. But a pH and blood gas analysis will rule it out completely. The pH was 7.58 (alkaline), PCO_2 was 50 mm., PO_2 was 85 mm. (normal) excluding pulmonary emphysema with respiratory acidosis (Table 5). A history of repeated vomiting for the past 48 hours given by the family plus a subsequent barium swallow made the diagnosis of *pyloric obstruction* (see page 99). In retrospect it is very possible to have a normal plasma sodium concentration in this condition since gastric juice contains water in excess of sodium (only 50 mEq. of $Na^+/L.$) compared to plasma. Yet total body sodium would be depleted.

Diagnostic Problems—Case 2

J.L. was a 16-year-old white female brought to the emergency room in coma. Her admission electrolytes were:

Na—151 mEq./L.
K—3.2 mEq./L.
Cl—120 mEq./L.
HCO_3^-—9 mEq./L.

Turning to Table 2 there is no pattern like this among the common disorders, but salicylate intoxication and acute renal failure are the closest to it. The high sodium and chloride would suggest severe dehydration and indeed that was the case clinically. Calculation of the serum osmolality can be done to prove it.

$$mOsm./L. = (Na + K) \times (1.9) + \frac{FBS}{18} + \frac{BUN}{2.8}$$

or roughly $2 \times (Na + K) = 308$

This is high (normal 270-290). Significant dehydration is not usually found in early salicylate intoxication or renal failure. Looking at the most striking feature of the electrolytes there must be something

else going on since the bicarbonate is extremely low. Table 3 shows that a low bicarbonate is increasingly found in salicylate intoxication, diabetic acidosis, renal tubular acidosis, renal failure and other forms of metabolic acidosis. Simple calculation for a significant anion gap should make one suspicious of diabetic or lactic acidosis using the following formula:

Anion gap = $(Na + K) - (Cl + HCO_3^-)$
Anion gap = $(151 + 3.2) - (120 + 9)$
Anion gap = 25.2 (normal = 12 ± 4)

The anion gap is high. Thus diabetic or lactic acidosis must be highly suspected. Examining the patient clinically for hyperpnea would be of little help since it is seen in all the conditions mentioned. However, a blood pH would be very helpful. Blood gas studies revealed a pH of 6.73 (which is extremely unusual in a live patient) a PCO_2 of 32 mm. and an HCO_3^- of 10. Thus salicylate intoxication is ruled out because the pH is usually high until later in the illness or unless extremely large doses have been ingested giving enough hydrogen ion to cause a metabolic acidosis. The blood glucose of 453 mg. percent and a serum acetone positive to 1:20 (dilution) clinched the diagnosis of *diabetic acidosis* (see page 133).

This case illustrates that while the total body sodium and chloride are invariably reduced in diabetic acidosis, if body water is lost in excess of sodium and chloride the plasma concentration of both may be increased.

Diagnostic Problems—Case 3

J.L. was a 67-year-old, alert, white male who had admission electrolytes of:

Na—127 mEq./L.
K—4.1 mEq./L.
Cl—90 mEq./L.
HCO_3^-—31 mEq./L.

Table 2 shows no disease which typically presents with a pattern of low sodium, normal potassium, low chloride and slightly elevated bicarbonate. However pulmonary emphysema and congestive heart failure present with two out of three of these abnormalities. Table 4 indicates that in addition to the above disorders, diuretics (mercurials especially), inappropriate ADH secretion, excessive sweating and pyloric obstruction may also resemble this picture. A metabolic acidosis such as diabetic ketosis is unlikely to present with such a high bicarbonate. Chronic renal failure is unlikely for the same reason. It is also unlikely that there is a laboratory error since the anion gap is 10 (normal = 12 ± 4). Clinically there was a history of chronic congestive heart failure and pulmonary emphysema. Also the patient had been on diuretics (Aldactone and Lasix). There was no history of vomiting or ulcer. Pulmonary emphysema was ruled out as a significant problem here by normal arterial PCO_2 and pH, (7.45) (Table 5). The question was whether the patient had lost enormous amounts of salt (in excess of water) and water from the diuretics or was still retaining salt and water (in excess of salt) despite the use of the diuretics. Serum osmolality was 248 mOsm./Kg., but this merely confirmed the existence of hyponatremia. The urine osmolality was 272 mOsm/Kg. which is extremely low and suggests sodium retention. A low plasma albumin and hematocrit also suggested that the condition was dilutional hyponatremia due to severe congestive heart failure (page 89). Thus his total body sodium was actually increased. A blood volume was performed and found to be markedly increased, confirming the diagnosis.

Diagnostic Problems—Case 4

Admission electrolytes on this 86-year-old white male were:

Na—150 mEq./L.
K—5.0 mEq./L.
Cl—114 mEq./L.
HCO_3^-—15 mEq./L.

At a glance the electrolytes suggest dehydration and an acid-base disorder. Table 2 fails to show a pattern of this nature among the common diseases. Table 3 shows that hypernatremia may result from dehydration, pathologic diaphoresis, diabetes insipidus, primary aldosteronism and administration of normal saline or hypertonic saline I.V. A low bicarbonate rules out primary aldosteronism (Table 2) and there was no history of intervenous fluid administration. Table 4 suggests that in addition to the above possibilities diabetic acidosis with dehydration, acute renal insufficiency with dehydration and salicylate intoxication may produce this picture. Indeed the patient showed mushy eyeballs, tenting of the skin and dry tongue clinically confirming the dehydration. Calculation of the anion gap was done with the following formula:

Anion gap = $(Na + K) - (Cl + HCO_3^-)$
Anion gap = $(150 + 5) - (114 + 15)$
Anion gap = 26
(Normal = 12 ± 4)

So the anion gap was at least 10 above normal. Ketones of diabetes or starvation might explain this. Indeed the patient's blood sugar was 424 mg percent. High phosphates and sulfates of renal insufficiency might also explain this. The BUN and creatinine were both markedly elevated. The patient died before serum acetone and pH could be determined and so one is forced to conclude that the patient had *dehydration* (page 77) with probable *diabetic acidosis* (page 133) and *acute renal insufficiency* (page 107).

This case illustrates that many clinical problems in electrolyte metabolism are due to two or more coexistent diseases.

Diagnostic Problems—Case 5

A 65-year-old, white male had the following admission electrolytes:

Na—141 mEq./L.
K—3.1 mEq./L.
Cl—83 mEq./L.
HCO_3^-—47 mEq./L.

Table 2 indicates that primary aldosteronism and pulmonary emphysema may show this pattern. In addition pyloric obstruction is compatible with three

out of four of these abnormalities. Since both *primary aldosteronism* and *pyloric obstruction* would present with an *alkalosis* while *pulmonary emphysema* would present with an *acidosis,* a pH and blood gas analysis are crucial in differentiating the three. Arterial blood gas analysis revealed a pH of 7.27, Po_2 of 51 mm. and Pco_2 of 67 mm. Hg. Table 5 shows this pattern is typical of pulmonary emphysema. Clinically the patient was lethargic, hyperventilating and the family related that he had a long history of respiratory problems and was a heavy smoker. This confirmed the diagnosis.

Diagnostic Problems—Case 6

A 56-year-old, white female diabetic had the following admission electrolytes:

Na—120 mEq./L.
K—3.5 mEq./L.
Cl—68 mEq./L.
HCO_3^-—36 mEq./L.

Here fasting blood sugar and serum acetone were normal. The sodium and chloride are markedly reduced, the potassium is low normal and the bicarbonate is high. These would suggest either salt depletion or dilutional hyponatremia with a metabolic alkalosis or respiratory acidosis. Table 2 indicates that pyloric obstruction and pulmonary emphysema, as well as *excessive use of diuretics,* may resemble this picture. Table 4 suggests that in addition to the above *pulmonary emphysema* with *congestive heart failure* and *diabetic acidosis* with pulmonary em-

physema may have similar findings. Blood gases ruled out pulmonary emphysema (Table 5) as a cause of the bicarbonate elevation as they revealed a pH of 7.54 (alkalosis), a Pco_2 of 38 mm. and a Po_2 of 69 mm. There was no history of vomiting or diarrhea.

Clinical examination was the key to the differential diagnosis. There were mushy eyeballs, dry tongue, loss of skin turgor—all signs of dehydration. A serum albumin and hematocrit were high and confirmed the volume depletion. A blood volume would be more specific. However, since the serum sodium and chloride are usually high in dehydration there must be chronic salt-losing nephritis or excessive diuretic therapy to explain the salt depletion along with the volume depletion. Old clinic records confirmed the suspicion that the patient was on *heavy doses of diuretics.* She was taking furosemide 40 mg. q.i.d. and Aldactazide one tablet q.i.d. Discontinuing the medication and providing a normal fluid and electrolyte intake restored the electrolytes to normal.

Diagnostic Problems—Case 7

C.M. is a 44-year-old, white female with the following electrolyte results on admission:

Na—128 mEq./L.
K—2.6 mEq./L.
Cl—91 mEq./L.
HCO_3^-—3 mEq./L.

Since the patient was not unconscious and a huge anion gap of 36.6 was calculated using the formula on page 162 a laboratory error was assumed and the electrolytes were repeated. However, the results were practically the same. A look at Table 2 indicates that diabetic acidosis, diarrhea of whatever cause, prolonged use of diuretics and chronic renal failure are common conditions that may produce this pic-

ture. Table 4 shows that in addition to the above, lactic acidosis may produce a similar picture. The history revealed that she was not a known diabetic, but she had been taking furosemide 60 mg. a day for some time. There was no history of diarrhea. The fasting blood sugar was normal but a BUN was 206 mg. percent, the creatinine was 13.1 mg. percent and the phosphates were 13.4 mg. percent (accounting partially for the anion gap). Urine output the first 24 hours was only 300 ml. All this supported a diagnosis of chronic renal failure with acute exacerbation, but the fact that the BUN was much more than 10 times the creatinine suggested that there was also prerenal azotemia due to either congestive heart failure, dehydration or shock. Blood pressure and central venous pressure were normal and since she had been on furosemide it was felt that *dehydration* was partially due to that. Loading her with 3,000 ml. of a balanced electrolyte solution and two ampules of sodium bicarbonate (89.2 mEq.) produced marked clinical improvement, an increase in her urine output

Diagnostic Problems—Case 8

A 56 year-old, white female diabetic was admitted with mild epigastic pain, nausea and occasional vomiting. Admission electrolytes were:

Na—131 mEq./L.
K—3.4 mEq./L.
Cl—91 mEq./L.
HCO_3^-—24 mEq./L.

Calculation of the anion gap (formula on page 162) revealed only a slight elevation but the BUN, creatinine and serum acetone were normal although her fasting blood sugar was 225 mg. percent. Her pH was 7.38. An upper G.I. series was done and revealed a small duodenal ulcer. She was put on a progressive Sippy diet, and an I.V. of 5 percent dextrose and water was started with a "keep open" order.

Five days after admission the patient became confused and irritable and the resident was called. Electrolytes were ordered and revealed the following:

Na—104 mEq./L.
K—4.2 mEq./L.
Cl—70 mEq./L.
HCO_3^-—24 mEq./L.

The serum acetone was negative and the fasting blood sugar was 125 mg. percent.

Diagnostic Problems—Case 9

An elderly white male was admitted to the hospital with the following electrolyte results:

Na—161 mEq./L.
K—6.6 mEq./L.
Cl—125 mEq./L.
HCO_3^-—13 mEq./L.

Table 2 does not show this pattern to be typical of the common electrolyte disorders, but acute renal failure is associated with three out of four of these abnormalities (high potassium, high chloride, low bicarbonate). Calculation of the anion gap (using formula on page 162) shows it to be abnormally high (approximately 30) so that a *laboratory error* was considered. However, repeat electrolytes were the same.

and a drop in the BUN. It was concluded that her problem was a combination of *renal failure* and *dehydration* (from the diuretics).

Table 2 shows that untreated congestive heart failure is a common cause of this alteration. However, there was no clinical evidence of this. Table 4 shows that in addition, chronic renal failure, excessive sweating, certain diuretics, inappropriate ADH secretion and excessive intake of water without electrolytes may present this picture. Reviewing the chart the resident found that on the "keep open" order the patient had received an average of 2,500 ml. of fluid (without electrolytes) a day. In addition oral intake of food was poor and she had vomited at least twice a day. For two days prior to the onset of confusion she had a total of 10 loose stools. These undoubtedly balanced the alkalotic effect of the vomiting and left her with a dilutional hyponatremia from *excessive intake of water without electrolytes*. This case illustrates that when fluids are ordered to keep a vein open they must include electrolytes if they are to be continued for any length of time. Also one should specify how many drops a minute the I.V. should run. Although 25 to 35 drops a minute may seem slow, this could deliver 120 ml. an hour or 2,900 ml. a day. Running an I.V. at less than 16 drops a minute (1 ml. a min.) may lead to clotting unless heparin is added to the I.V. solution. If it is desirable to keep a vein open for a long period it is wise to clamp and cut the tubing and inject heparin into the portion remaining to prevent clotting.

Diabetic acidosis, lactic acidosis and renal failure are the most common conditions associated with a large anion gap. Table 4 indicated that in addition to these conditions renal failure with severe dehydration, severe diarrhea, diabetic acidosis with severe dehydration and starvation with dehydration may produce this picture. The blood pH was 7.23 and supported the diagnosis of a metabolic acidosis. Clinically, there was tenting of the skin, mushy eyeballs and a dry coated tongue supporting a diagnosis of dehydration. The BUN was 260 mg. percent, the creatinine was 11 mg. percent and the phosphates were 7.1 mg. percent. Serum osmolality was 342 mOsm./Kg. (high) as expected with dehydration, but most remarkable was a urine osmolality of 364 mOsm./Kg. indicating that the kidneys could not concentrate the urine and supporting the diagnosis of *renal failure*. After 3,000 ml. of 5 percent dextrose and water daily over the next three days the electrolytes were:

    Na—135 mEq./L.
    K—5.4 mEq./L.
    Cl—106 mEq./L.
    HCO_3^-—16 mEq./L.

Diagnostic Problems—Case 10

A 51-year-old, white male was admitted to the hospital with a history of headache, vomiting once or twice a day and papilledema. Angiography revealed a large posterior fossa tumor. His admission electrolytes were:

    Na—142 mEq./L.
    K—4.2 mEq./L.
    Cl—96 mEq./L.
    HCO_3^-—28 mEq./L.

Following angiography he did not take much food or drink for five days and vomited occasionally. Then he developed a sudden increase of vomiting to six or seven times a day. Electrolytes at this time were:

    Na—140 mEq./L.
    K—6.0 mEq./L.
    Cl—96 mEq./L.
    HCO_3^-—25 mEq./L.

The only major alteration in this electrolyte picture is hyperkalemia. A look at Table 3 shows that acute renal failure, certain diuretics (e.g., spironolactone), adrenal insufficiency and acidosis are most likely to cause this picture.

He was not on diuretics and with a normal bicarbonate acidosis is unlikely. Furthermore vomiting should produce an alkalosis and hypokalemia. However, the anion gap (calculated by using the formula on page 162) is 25. Therefore, he must have an increase in either ketones, or phosphates and sulfates, or lactic acid. The pH was 7.28. To explain the combination of hyperkalemia, acidosis with a significant anion gap, and a normal bicarbonate one must postulate that the patient has more than one disorder. His BUN was 80 mg. percent and his creatinine was 6.2 mg. percent. Acute renal failure would explain the hyperkalemia, but not the normal sodium and bicarbonate. An upper G.I. series showed *pyloric obstruction* and so this explained the normal bicarbonate. A serum protein was high and a blood volume was low so that this explained the normal sodium in the face of acute renal failure. He was *dehydrated*.

This case demonstrates once again that many clinical disorders of fluid and electrolyte balance are a combination of two or more conditions.

The BUN had dropped to 207 mg. percent but the creatinine did not change. This was further evidence of primary *renal failure with dehydration*.

This case illustrates once again that combinations of two or more disorders may be responsible for the electrolyte derangements. Such situations are common and must be looked for.

TREATMENT PROBLEMS

Treatment Problems—Case 1

J.L. was admitted with the following admission laboratory results:

> Na—151 mEq./L.
> K—3.2 mEq./L.
> Cl—120 mEq./L.
> HCO_3^-—9 mEq./L.
> Glucose—453 mg.%
> BUN—20 mg.%
> Serum acetone—positive in a dilution of 1:20

A diagnosis of diabetic acidosis was made. The patient weighed 60 Kg. The following electrolytes and solution were administered in addition to adequate amounts of insulin.

Immediately—	2 ampules of sodium bicarbonate I.V. (44.6 mEq./amp.)
First 2 Hours—	1,000 ml. of 0.45 normal saline with 40 mEq. of potassium chloride added and 600 ml. of 5 percent dextrose and 0.45 normal saline with 60 mEq. of potassium chloride.
Next 4 Hours—	1,000 ml. of 5 percent of dextrose and 0.45 normal saline with 60 mEq. potassium chloride.
Next 3½ Hours—	300 ml. of 5 percent dextrose and normal saline with 40 mEq. of potassium chloride; 500 ml. of dextrose and 0.45 normal saline with two ampules of sodium bicarbonate and 30 mEq. potassium chloride.

Thus she received a total of 3,400 ml. of fluid, approximately 180 mEq. of sodium bicarbonate, 290 mEq. of sodium chloride, and 230 mEq. of potassium chloride in the first 9½ hours.

Electrolytes repeated at the end of the above therapy revealed:

> Na—151 mEq./L.
> K—3.7 mEq./L.
> Cl—125 mEq./L.
> HCO_3^-—19 mEq./L.

Urine output was good.

How would you have treated the patient during the first 10 hours, if any different?

Answer. The patient had diabetic acidosis, but in addition was severely dehydrated.

Error 1

The bicarbonate deficit was not calculated. Using the formula on page 156:

$$\text{Bicarbonate deficit} = 25 - 9 \times 0.4 \times 60$$

$$\text{or}$$

$$\text{Bicarbonate deficit} = 384 \text{ mEq.}$$

Half of this should have been given during the first two hours and then the electrolytes and blood gases reassessed.

Error 2

This patient needed water more than electrolytes and lots of it. Therefore a 0.45 saline solution was a good choice, but 20 mEq. of potassium chloride in each bottle would have been adequate and kept it significantly hypotonic. She should have received at least 1,000 ml. an hour of this for the first five hours.

Error 3

Dextrose was given too soon (during the first two hours). It is unlikely that the sugar (453 mg.%) would have dropped so quickly.

Error 4

The calculated potassium deficit (using formula on page 156) was only 31.2 mEq. to start with. Therefore she probably received entirely too much potassium, although her good urine output kept her out of trouble.

Treatment Problems—Case 2

C.J. was an 80-year-old white female admitted for amputation of a gangrenous right leg. Her admission laboratory tests gave the following electrolyte results:

Na—135 mEq./L.
K—3.8 mEq./L.
Cl—105 mEq./L.
HCO_3^-—25 mEq./L.

These were considered to be within normal limits. Additional pertinent laboratory studies were fasting blood sugar of 175 mg. percent, BUN of 10 mg. percent and creatinine of 1.7 mg. percent. Thus her renal function was relatively good for her age. Nevertheless, it was felt prudent to begin a 24-hour intake and output recording from her first hospital day. She received an average of 1,300 ml. of fluids in the form of Vivonex for the first five days. She went into mild shock on the sixth hospital day and surgery was cancelled. Electrolytes at that time were:

Na—134 mEq./L.
K—3.6 mEq./L.
Cl—99 mEq./L.
HCO_3^-—31 mEq./L.

These were considered normal. For the next three days she received an average of 2,500 ml. per day of fluid in the form of 5 percent dextrose and 0.2 normal saline with 10 mEq. of potassium chloride in each liter bottle. Surgery was done on the ninth hospital day. On the day of surgery she received 2,000 ml. of 5 percent dextrose in Ringer's lactate. Then the intravenous infusions were discontinued. Her urine output during this time averaged 900 ml. a day. The first 2 days after the intravenous fluids were discontinued she took 1,000 ml. of fluid a day orally. However for the next 6 days her oral intake was practically nothing despite an average urine output of 600 ml. a day. Electrolytes at the end of this period were:

Na—151 mEq./L.
K—3.8 mEq./L.
Cl—111 mEq./L.
CO_2—30

In addition her BUN had risen to 45 mg. percent. The clinicians rightly concluded that she was dehydrated and began intravenous fluids again. For the next three days she received an average of 2,300 ml. of I.V. fluids a day mostly 5 percent dextrose with 20 to 30 mEq. of potassium chloride in every 1,000 ml.

Urine output averaged 1,300 ml. a day. At the end of this period electrolytes were:

Na—146 mEq./L.
K—3.6 mEq./L.
Cl—103 mEq./L.
HCO_3^-—35 mEq./L.

The clinicians interpreted the slight elevation of the sodium as a need for more fluids and the high bicarbonate as a laboratory error. The next three days she received an average of 4,300 ml. of fluids a day in the form of 5 percent dextrose and 0.2 or 0.45 normal saline with 20 mEq. of potassium chloride in each bottle of 1,000 ml. Her urine output averaged 2,500 ml. a day during this period. She promptly went into congestive heart failure. Her electrolytes at this time were:

Na—127 mEq./L.
K—3.4 mEq./L.
Cl—90 mEq./L.
HCO_3^-—30 mEq./L.

What was more significant was that her serum albumin had dropped from 3.5 to 2.5 gm. and her BUN had risen to 33 mg. percent.

What were the errors in the management of this patient? What was the proper management?

Error 1

Total intake of fluid during the first five days was inadequate (1,200 ml./day) accounting for the shock at the time surgery was first planned. Yet the serum electrolyte concentrations were not much changed from the time of admission. This is because electrolyte replacement was also inadequate. 1,200 ml. of Vivonex contains only 45 mEq. of sodium (30 mEq. less than the daily requirement), 36 mEq. of potassium (14 mEq. less than the daily requirement) and 60 mEq. of chloride (17 mEq. less than the daily requirements). She should have received at least 1,600 ml. of fluid a day. This could have been Vivonex (standard diet) provided adequate electrolyte replacement also was given.

Error 2

Total intake of fluid for the first eight days postoperatively was 2,000 ml. Insensible water loss alone would require 800 ml. a day or 6,400 ml. during this period leading to a deficit of 4,400 ml. In addition with a urine output of 600 ml. a day she developed a deficit of 4,800 ml. more bringing her total deficit to 9,200 ml. Catabolism may have produced 200 ml. of water a day reducing the deficit to 7,600 ml. Proper management would have been to give her at least 1,500 ml. of fluid a day or a total of 9,000 ml. postoperatively to allow for good urine output and some sensible (sweat) water loss. This should have been in the form of 1,000 ml. of 5 percent dextrose with 20 mEq. of potassium chloride, and 500 ml. of normal saline with 20 mEq. of potassium chloride.

Error 3

Once the severe dehydration was discovered treatment was inadequate the first three days (2,300 ml. a day with a 1,300 ml. urine output), but was excessive the next three days leading to congestive heart failure. Treatment of moderate dehydration in the normal adult should be 2,400 ml./square meter of body surface. Referring to Table 8, a 60 Kg. adult who is 5 feet 5 inches tall has a surface area of 1.65 sq. m. Thus she normally might need 1.65 × 2,400 or 3,960 ml. a day in the beginning. However because of her age, cautious reevaluation after two or three days of this therapy to include body weight, intake and output, blood volume and serum and urine osmolality would have indicated the need for a reduction to approximately 3,000 ml. a day. One might question this evaluation because she put out 2,500 ml. of urine a day while on 4,300 ml. of fluid a day. However her high urine output was partly due to a solute diuresis from her diabetes (FBS was 300 to 400 mg. percent during this period). It is also evident that she had mild renal insufficiency (BUN was 33 mg. percent) and so her kidneys may have had poor concentration power. One should remember that it is difficult to calculate daily fluid requirement from the urine output in patients with chronic renal insufficiency.

Treatment Problems—Case 3

A 75-year-old Negro male was admitted to the hospital with the following initial electrolyte results:

Na—159 mEq./L.
K—4.4 mEq./L.
Cl—127 mEq./L.
HCO_3^-—25 mEq./L.

Calculation of the anion gap (formula on page 162) revealed it to be normal so that a laboratory error was not suspected. Table 2 reveals that *dehydration* and *diabetes insipidus* may produce this picture. The serum osmolality was 332 mOsm./Kg. whereas the urine osmolality was 735 mOsm./Kg. This ruled out diabetes insipidus (page 119). The clinical picture was consistent with *severe dehydration*. The patient was treated with 2,000 to 3,000 ml. of 5 percent dextrose daily for the next six days after which the following electrolyte results were obtained:

Na—138 mEq./L.
K—4.7 mEq./L.
Cl—106 mEq./L.
HCO_3^-—36 mEq./L.

BUN and creatinine were normal and the urine output had been 1,500 ml. a day.

Question 1

Was the treatment proper? No! Normal individuals lose 40 to 50 mEq. potassium a day and this patient did not have that replaced. However an elderly man such as this may lose as much as a third of his renal function (without an elevation of the BUN or creatinine) from arteriosclerosis. Therefore, possibly 20 to 30 mEq. potassium would have been adequate replacement of losses.

Question 2

Why did his serum potassium remain normal? Part of this could be due to the mild renal insufficiency, but there must have been other factors. Since he only received 100 to 150 gm. of glucose a day (allowing him only 400-600 calories a day) he must have relied on tissue catabolism for energy. This would release moderate amounts of potassium. He may also have had a mild adrenal insufficiency preventing the drop in potassium (Table 1). Finally the high bicarbonate may indicate that he had pulmonary emphysema with associated respiratory acidosis. This would cause potassium to move out of the cell in exchange for hydrogen ion. Blood gas analysis would determine this.

Treatment Problems—Case 4

A 72-year-old, comatose Negro male was admitted to the hospital with the following initial electrolyte results:

Na—128 mEq./L.   Cl—100 mEq./L.
K—6.4 mEq./L. HCO_3^-—13 mEq./L.

The anion gap (formula on page 162) was slightly elevated (21.4). However repeat electrolytes were almost the same so that a laboratory error was excluded. There are no conditions in Table 2 with this pattern, but *acute renal failure* presents with at least three of these alterations. Indeed the patient had a BUN of 71 mg. percent, a creatinine of 2.4 mg. percent and a uric acid of 12 mg. percent. Table 4 shows that in addition to acute renal failure, diabetic acidosis with renal failure and acute acidosis from any cause may produce this picture (potassium shifts out of the cell in exchange for hydrogen ion). The patient's blood sugar was 1,425 mg. percent and the serum acetone was strongly positive in a dilution of 1:4, clinching the diagnosis of *diabetic acidosis* with *acute renal failure*.

Therapy was begun with insulin and intravenous fluids. The first 24 hours the patient received 2,000 ml. of 5 percent dextrose and 1,000 ml. of normal saline with 44.6 mEq. sodium bicarbonate. He only had 400 ml. urine output. He received a total of 110 units of regular insulin and 50 units of NPH insulin. At the end of this period he was alert but a bit confused. Electrolytes were:

Na—133 mEq./L.   Cl—93 mEq./L.
K—4.4 mEq./L. HCO_3^-—26 mEq./L.

The blood sugar was 550 mg. percent. An 1,800 calorie ADA diet was begun. He received 3,000 ml. of normal saline and 1,000 ml. of 5 percent dextrose the next 24 hours, together with a total of 80 units of insulin. His urine output rose to 1,900 ml. and he was almost completely recovered clinically. Electrolytes at this point were:

Na—136 mEq./L.   Cl—93 mEq./L.
K—2.8 mEq./L. HCO_3^-—28 mEq./L.

Blood sugar was 280 mg. percent. BUN, creatinine and uric acid were normal. He received 3,000 ml. of 5 percent dextrose with 20 units of regular insulin in each bottle of 1,000 ml. during the next 24 hours and then the intravenous fluids were discontinued. He was discharged three days later on an 1,800 calorie ADA diet and 30 units of NPH insulin daily. His physician was pleased with the clinical results.

What would you have done differently?

Error 1

Electrolytes were done only once every 24 hours. They should be done every two or three hours, at least during the first day.

Error 2

In most cases of diabetic acidosis at least 4 to 6 liters of fluid must be given the first 8 to 24 hours. However the age and the complication of acute renal failure possibly prompted this clinician to give much less. Nevertheless, if a central venous pressure line had been inserted the treatment could have been more vigorous.

Error 3

Very little bicarbonate was given. With more frequent monitoring of electrolytes and pH more could have been given, but the outcome would have been the same. Calculation of the deficit may be made by the following formula:

$$HCO_3^- \text{ deficit} = \text{body weight in Kg.} \times 0.4$$
$$\times (\text{desired } [HCO_3^-]$$
$$- \text{measured } [HCO_3^-])$$
$$\text{or}$$
$$HCO_3^- \text{ deficit} = 60 \times .4 \times (25-13)$$
$$= 24 \times 12$$
$$= 288 \text{ mEq. of NaHCO}_3$$

Usually 50 percent of this is given initially and the electrolytes and pH are determined in two to four hours to see if more is needed.

Error 4

Therapy is usually begun with normal saline rather than 5 percent dextrose. Since the plasma is hypertonic 0.45 normal saline is often given after the first bottle of normal saline.

Error 5

Too little insulin was given. Most standard treatment programs for diabetic acidosis call for 50 to 100 units of regular insulin IV and 50 units subcutaneously initially and at least 50 units every two to three hours after that until a good response is noted. A report in Lancet (2:515, 1973) suggests that 5 to 20 units of regular insulin I.M. hourly may be just as adequate. However, frequent monitoring of the blood sugar, BUN and electrolytes must be done.

Error 6

No potassium was given intravenously. There is a tremendous shift of potassium out of the cells in exchange for hydrogen ion in diabetic acidosis. This is excreted in the urine. This must be replaced during therapy especially since insulin and glucose take a lot of potassium with them into the cell. This patient did not show a low serum potassium until later because

of the associated renal failure. When it did show, 50 to 75 mEq. should have been given and the electrolytes rechecked.

Treatment Problems—Case 5

A 60-year-old white female was admitted with a history of vomiting coffee-ground material for nine days. Her admission electrolytes were:

Na—140 mEq./L.   Cl—87 mEq./L.
K—3.2 mEq./L. HCO_3^-—40 mEq./L.

A BUN was 37 mg. percent and creatinine was 2.1 mg. percent. Aside from the normal sodium these were the electrolytes to be expected in pyloric or upper intestinal obstruction. An upper G.I. series confirmed the presence of a pyloric ulcer. Gastric analysis revealed 55 mEq. of free acid per liter. A nasogastric tube was inserted and intravenous therapy begun. In preparation for surgery she received an average of 3,500 ml. of fluid a day most of which was 5 percent dextrose and 0.5 normal saline. She also received an average of 90 mEq. of potassium a day. Her output from the nasogastric tube averaged approximately 1,000 ml. a day while her urine output averaged 1,800 ml. a day. By the fifth hospital day she had the following electrolytes:

Na—135 mEq./L.   Cl—99 mEq./L.
K—6.3 mEq./L. HCO_3^-—27 mEq./L.

Her BUN and creatinine had returned to normal. What accounted for these electrolyte changes?

Answer. She was given entirely too much potassium. Gastric juice with a high free acid (which she had) contains only 10 mEq. of potassium per liter. She excreted a liter a day via this route. The potassium in this plus approximately 40 mEq. of potassium obligatory loss in the urine would necessitate a maintenance dose of only 50 mEq. a day. Replacement of her losses prior to admission could be calculated by the following formula.

$$\text{Potassium deficit} = \text{Desired serum potassium} - \text{present serum potassium} \times \text{double the extracellular volume}[17]$$

This lady weighed 60 Kg. so her extracellular volume is 12 liters. Double that is 24 liters.

$$\text{Her potassium deficit} = 4.5 - 3.2 \times 24$$
$$\text{or} \qquad 31.2 \text{ mEq.}$$

So on the first day approximately 81 mEq. of potassium would have been adequate and she needed only 50 mEq. daily subsequently.

Treatment Problems—Case 6

A 45-year-old white male underwent a vagotomy and pyloroplasty. He received 2,000 ml. of 5 percent dextrose and water the day of the operation. He had 1,200 ml. of urine output during that period and 1,000 ml. of fluid was removed by nasogastric suction.

Question. What should be his fluid and electrolyte prescription for the next 24 hours?

1. Total fluid for the next 24 hours should equal urine output plus insensible water loss plus losses by nasogastric suction, or 1,200 + 800 + 1,000 = 3,000 ml.

2. Since 1,000 ml. of this is gastric juice a look at Table 6 shows that this is best replaced with 0.5 normal saline and 20 mEq. of potassium chloride.

3. Since his urine output was good he probably lost an additional 40 to 60 mEq. of potassium in the urine.

4. The effects of surgery on sodium retention are probably still active (page 153) so the remaining fluid requirements should be replaced with 5 percent dextrose and water.

Thus he will receive:

1st bottle: 1,000 ml. of 5 percent dextrose and water with 20 mEq. potassium chloride.

2nd bottle: 1,000 ml. of N/2 saline with 20 mEq. of potassium chloride added.

3rd bottle: 1,000 ml. of 5 percent dextrose and water with 20 mEq. of potassium chloride added.

Treatment Problems—Case 7

A 12-year-old white male suffered third degree burns to his entire left forearm and the anterior surface of his trunk. If he weighed 40 Kg. what are his fluid and electrolyte requirements for the first 24 hours?

Answer. Using the rule of nines he has one half of an upper extremity or 4½ percent and the anterior trunk or 18 percent for a total of 22 or 23 percent. His requirements are (See formula, page 139):

1. Plasma 0.5 ml. $\times$ 23 $\times$ 40 = 460 ml.

2. Ringer's lactate = 1.5 ml. $\times$ 23 $\times$ 40
   = 1,380 ml.
3. Basic needs = 1,500 ml. 5 percent dextrose and water

Since less than 30 percent of his body was burned 1,000 ml. of Ringer's lactate would be given followed by the 460 ml. of plasma in the first eight hours. Then 1,000 ml. of 5 percent dextrose and water would be given in the next eight hours and 380 ml. of Ringer's lactate and 500 ml. of 5 percent dextrose and water in the final eight hours.

Treatment Problems—Case 8

A 78-year-old white female was transferred from a nursing home because of failure to take much food or drink for five days. Admission electrolytes were:

Na—159 mEq./L.
K—4.0 mEq./L.
Cl—120 mEq./L.
HCO_3^-—28 mEq./L.

A diagnosis of severe dehydration was made. What is her water deficit if she weighed 55 Kg. prior to the illness?

Using the formula on page 156:

$$\text{Body water deficit} = \frac{\text{measured Na} - \text{ideal Na}}{\text{ideal Na}}$$
$$\times \text{ normal body water}$$

Normal body water = 0.6
$$\times \text{ normal body wt. in Kg.}$$

Normal body water = 33 liters

$$\text{Deficit} = \frac{159 - 138}{138} \times 33 \text{ liters}$$

Deficit = 5.02 liters

If her weight prior to the illness was not known, her present weight could be used to calculate the deficit and then repeat electrolytes would determine additional needs.

Treatment Problems—Case 9

A three-month-old infant developed moderate diarrhea (12-15 stools a day). His admission weight was 6 Kg. On his last visit to the office two weeks before, he had weighed 7.5 Kg. What fluid would be administered and how much?

Answer. As stated on page 101, a good intravenous prescription for this infant is 5 percent dextrose and N/3 saline with 20 mEq. of potassium chloride and ½ ampule (22.3 mEq.) of sodium bicarbonate

added. Inosol B with 5 percent dextrose (page 158) could also be used. The deficit is based on his normal weight (7.5 Kg.) minus his present weight (6 Kg.) or 1.5 Kg. He needs 1,500 ml. of the above formula plus his maintenance for the next 24 hours which would be 1,500 ml./sq. m. of body surface or 1,500 $\times$ .39 (see Table 8) in his case. This would be 585 ml. A good pediatric maintenance fluid is N/4 saline and 5 percent dextrose (see Table 7) with 20 mEq. of potassium chloride per liter added.

Treatment Problems—Case 10

A 46-year-old white male was admitted with a five-day history of vomiting six or seven times a day and very little intake. His admission electrolytes were:

Na—134 mEq./L.   Cl—74 mEq./L.
K—2.5 mEq./L. HCO_3^-—56 mEq./L.

Blood ph was 7.55. Upper G.I. series revealed a pyloric ulcer with obstruction. What would be his fluid and electrolyte prescription for the first 24 hours if his body weight is 80 Kg.?

Answer. The first step is to calculate the chloride and potassium deficits using the formulas on page 156.

Chloride Deficit

Chloride deficit = ideal chloride (100) − measured chloride × 0.2 × body weight in Kg.

Chloride deficit = $100 - 74 \times 0.2 \times 80$

Chloride deficit = 416 mEq.

Table 6 shows that gastric juice contains 90 to 155 mEq. of chloride per liter so that this man has lost at least 3 to 4 liters of gastric juice to reach this chloride deficit. Thus 3.5 liters of N/2 saline with 20 mEq. of potassium chloride in each liter (the replacement fluid of choice listed in Table 6) should be given. To be sure this replaces the potassium, that deficit should be calculated separately.

Potassium Deficit

$$\text{Potassium deficit} = \text{ideal K (4.5)}$$
$$- 2.5 \times 0.40 \times 80$$
$$= 2.0 \times .40 \times 80$$
$$= 64 \text{ mEq.}$$

In 3.5 liters with 20 mEq. of potassium chloride per liter there would be 70 mEq. of potassium, which is only slightly more than he needs. Thus this solution would satisfy all the replacement of deficits pretty well.

Maintenance

This patient needs approximately 2,000 ml. of fluid for maintenance and as shown on page 157 this can be 1,000 ml. of 10 percent dextrose and water with 20 mEq. of potassium chloride added, 500 ml. of 10 percent dextrose and water with 10 mEq. of potassium chloride added, and 500 ml. of 5 percent dextrose and normal saline with 20 mEq. of potassium chloride added. Since all three of these solutions are hypertonic one should begin therapy with a liter of the replacement fluid and alternate with a liter or 500 ml. of one of these solutions.

Since a total of 5.5 liters must be given in 24 hours it is wise to calculate how much must be given each hour (approximately 230 ml. an hour in this case) and write this in the nursing orders. A "keep open" order of 5 percent dextrose and water should be written also to avoid the necessity of using a new vein.

References

1. Gamble, J. L.: Chemical Anatomy, Physiology, and Pathology of Extracellular Fluid. Cambridge, Harvard Univ. Press, 1949.
2. Maxwell, M. H. and Kleeman, C. R.: Clinical Disorders of Fluid and Electrolyte Metabolism. (ed. 2), New York, McGraw-Hill, 1972.
3. Sonnenblich, E. H., Cannon, P. J. and Laragh, J. H.: The nature of the action of intravenous aldosterone: evidence for a role of the hormone in urinary dilution. J. Clin. Invest., *40*:903, 1961.
4. Wilson, R. F.: Fluids, Electrolytes and Metabolism. Thomas, Springfield, Ill., 1973.
5. Filley, G. F.: Acid-Base and Blood Gas Regulation. Lea & Febiger, Philadelphia, 1971.
6. Selkurt, E. E.: Physiology. Little, Brown, Boston, 1963.
7. Collins, R. D.: Illustrated Manual of Laboratory Diagnosis. (ed. 2), Philadelphia, Lippincott, 1975.
8. Bondy, P. K.: Duncan's Diseases of Metabolism. (ed. 6), Philadelphia, Saunders, 1969.
9. Dirks, J. H., et al.: J. Clin. Invest., *44*:1160, 1965. The effects of saline infusion on sodium reabsorption by the proximal tubule of the dog.
10. Bland, J. H.: Clinical Metabolism of Body Water and Electrolytes. Philadelphia, Saunders, 1963.
11. Cannon, P. J., Ames, R. P. and Laragh, J. H.: Relation between potassium balance and aldosterone secretion in normal subjects and in patients with hypertensive or renal tubular disease. J. Clin. Invest., *45*:865, 1966.
12. Bergstrom, W. H.: The skeleton as an electrolyte reservoir. Metabolism, *5*:433, 1956.
13. Boedeker, E. C. and Danber J. H.: Manual of Medical Therapeutics. (ed. 21), Boston, Little, Brown, 1974.
14. Wintrobe, M. W., *et al.*: Harrison's Principles of Internal Medicine. (ed. 7), New York, McGraw-Hill, 1974.
15. Vertel, R. M. and Knochel, J. P.: Nonoliguric acute renal failure. JAMA, *200*:118, 1967.
16. Eliahou, H. E. and Bota, A.: The diagnosis of acute renal failure. Nephron, *2*:287, 1965.
17. Taylor, W. H.: Fluid Therapy and Disorders of Electrolyte Balance. Oxford, Blackwell, 1970.
18. Moore, F. D.: Tris buffer, mannitol and low viscus dextran. Surg. Clin. N. Amer., *43*:577, 1963.
19. Stanbury, J. B., Wyngaarden, J. B. and Fredrickson, D. S.: The Metabolic Basis of Inherited Disease (ed. 3), pp. 1548-1564. New York, McGraw-Hill, 1972.
20. Hillman, D. A., et al.: Renal (vasopressin-resistant) diabetes insipidus. Pediatrics, *21*:430, 1958.
21. Melby, J. C., *et al.*: Adrenal-Vein Catheterization of Localized Aldosterone-Producing Adenomas. New Engl. J. Med. *277*:1050, 1967.
22. Larcan, A., Huriet, C., Vert, P. and Thibant, G.: Non-acidiketosis metabolic comas in diabetics. Diabetes, *11*:99, 1963.
23. McCurdy, D. K.: Hyperosmolar Non-ketotic coma. Metab. Therapy, 3: No. 3, 1974.
24. Wolff, H. P. and Torbica, M.: Determination of plasma-aldosterone. Lancet, *2*:1346, 1963.
25. Beck, L. H. and Goldberg, M.: Diuretic therapy. Primary Care, *1*:165-178, 1974.
26. Goldberg, M.: The renal physiology of diuretics. *In* Orloff, J. and Berliner, R. W.: Handbook of Physiology, Sec. 8, Renal Physiology, pp. 1003-1031. Washington, D. C., 1973.
27. Fichman, M. P., *et al.*: Diuretic-induced hyponatremia. Ann. Intern. Med., *75*:853, 1971.
28. Weisberg, H. F.: Water, Electrolyte and Acid-Base Balance. (ed. 2), Baltimore, Williams & Wilkins, 1962.
29. Dubois, D. and Dubois, E. F.: Clinical calorimetry. Arch. Intern. Med., *17*:863, 1916.

Index